BOONE COUNTY LIBRARY
2040 9101 046 618 1

D0862351

Andra and Erin are the perfect pair of 40-somethings to lead us all to better awareness and health. With a combination of fact and fun, these two friends really have figured out the "fountain of youth."

~ Dr. Amina Shalash

Erin Smith is a master teacher. Erin weaves life lessons on how to show up fully present, how to be authentic, and how to love all of yourself. Through her devotion to yoga, Erin has impacted students' lives and through her new book, she has shared her powerful teachings on how to live healthily and happily.

~ Anella Wetter
M. Ed., RYT, Relationship Coach

Sensible Wellness For Women

Following the Four after the Big Four-Oh

Erin Smith, ERYT, CNT, MLS
Andra Sewalls, ERYT, CPT, MLS

Cork and Bottle Publishing

This book is written as a source of information only. The information contained in this book should by no means be considered a substitute for the advice of a qualified medical professional, who should always be consulted before beginning any new diet, exercise, or other health program.

All efforts have been made to ensure the accuracy of the information contained in this book as of the date published. The author(s) and the publisher expressly disclaim responsibility for any adverse effects arising from the use or application of the information herein.

Cork and Bottle books may be purchased for educational, business or sales promotional use. For information please write: Special Sales Department, Cork and Bottle Publishing, PO Box 910616, Lexington, KY 40591.

Book website: http://sensiblewellnessforwomen.com
Publisher website: http://corkandbottlepub.com
Author(s) website: http://theOMPlace.net

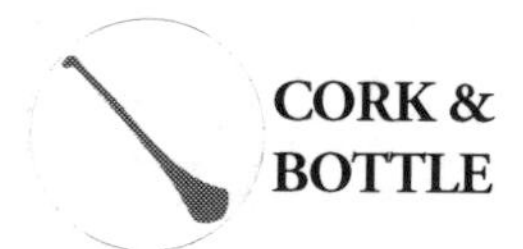

Cork and Bottle Publishing
Lexington, KY

FIRST EDITION
Published 2016

Library of Congress Cataloging-in-Publication Data is available upon request.

ISBN 978-0-692-67859-6

10 9 8 7 6 5 4 3 2 1

For our girls. May they always love themselves fiercely.

And for our bodies, who have served us lovingly, even when we took them for granted.

(Boring disclaimer) This publication contains the opinions and ideas of the authors. The reader should consult his or her own medical providers before adopting any of the suggestions in this book.

Hello, dear friend! We're so thrilled you took time out of your busy life to sit down with us for a bit. We understand how busy you are and what a challenge it is to carve out time to nurture yourself. We wrote this book because we know you want more and we can't wait to show you how to get it. We want to help you find self-love and empowerment and to let go of habits that are robbing you of your energy and natural beauty.

This is the one life we've been given and too many of us squander it trying to force our minds and bodies into unattainable ideals!

What does YOUR busy look like? Are you a wife? Mother? Boss? Sister? Daughter? Friend? Taking care of aging parents or grandkids? We get it! We really do. We've been in every one of those situations and let our health go as a result. Just like you, we have many people for whom we are responsible and often neglect ourselves as a result. We know who you are because we are you. Between us, we are wives, mothers, divorcees, entrepreneurs, sisters, daughters, pet owners, and friends. We aren't old enough to be grandparents yet, but our parents are in their 70s and need our help more and more.

At our age, we're concerned less with how we look than how we feel. We wouldn't trade the experience and wisdom we have now to be younger. We wouldn't swap our stretch marks, wrinkles or gray hair because they represent a life well lived. We don't want to look like we're 24. But we miss the energy we had at 24 and want that back. Yet the idea of taking on anything else can seem overwhelming.

But something compelled you to pick up this book. Maybe your hormones have gone berserk and your body is in "WTF" mode. Maybe your annual check-up results showed some less-than-awesome numbers, like high cholesterol or low bone density. Maybe you're losing your keys or forgetting appointments. Maybe you're having trouble sleeping or struggling to wake up and take on the world. Maybe you can no longer zip up a years-old favorite pair of jeans and it feels like losing a friend. We understand every one of these problems because they have all happened to us. The difference is that we refuse to accept these things as a natural result of the aging process.

Just like you, we were sick and tired of being sick and tired. Just like you, we knew that there was a better, more energetic us waiting to emerge. So we spent a decade figuring it out and want to share this news with you.

Your journey to complete wellness lies in making small changes each day. There is no beginning or end to health. True health and happiness is a cumulative effect of thousands of tiny decisions you make each day. We're here to suggest small ways you can start to encourage big change in your life. We will give you the tools and explain why and how you should use them to rediscover your vitality.

You are a naturally beautiful, radiant, and intelligent woman. But you probably don't notice this radiance because you are so tired and harried all the time. What if we told you that you can feel younger than your chronological age and have plenty of energy and fewer sick days? That you can finally become clear on what you want and who you want to be? That you can rediscover the joy of natural movement? And – this is our favorite part – that you can finally figure out how to rest and recover?

Are you ready to make the rest of your life the best of your life?

What is Wellness?

True wellness encompasses physical, mental, and spiritual health. When we were young, we were all taught to believe that health meant a thin, strong body. We now know it's so much more than that. Wellness is more than the mere elimination of symptoms. Wellness means adopting practices that will support the peak performance of your particular body, mind, and soul.

At our age, we have the experience to intuitively understand what works for us and what doesn't. The bad news is that we just don't have the time to give ourselves the attention we deserve. Jobs, spouses, children, pets, family, driving, and volunteering seem to eat up our days.

Think of your wellness as a bank account with every decision a deposit (like a long walk followed by yoga and meditation) or a withdrawal (like too much pizza washed down with too much beer). The body has an energy budget to spend but energy reserves are limited. Some body systems require more energy to run - if we spend too much energy in one place, we are forced to cut back on energy somewhere else to keep the budget balanced. It is up to us to decide how to best allocate our energy reserves to get the best return on our investments.

Wellness isn't about being perfect. It's about striking a balance between what you know and what you do.

Lifestyle diseases like heart disease, stroke, obesity, and diabetes now account for more deaths worldwide than infectious diseases. The World Health Organization (WHO) has projected that, by 2020, chronic diseases will account for more than three-quarters of all deaths worldwide. However, these so-called lifestyle diseases are almost entirely preventable. In 1900, your risk of being diagnosed with cancer was 1 in 30. In 2000, it was

1 in 2. At least 117 million Americans currently have a preventable, chronic disease. Just as troubling, surveys suggest fewer than half of American workers are satisfied with their jobs and a 2013 Harris poll indicates that only 1 in 3 Americans would call themselves "very happy".

We are clearly doing something fundamentally wrong. The solution has to start with us. What if we stopped making it harder on ourselves? What if we mindfully chose to give our bodies, minds, and souls what they needed to heal rather than relying on ineffective medical interventions?

Wolfing down a carton of ice cream because you had a bad day is disrespectful to your own awesomeness. Binge-watching Netflix night after night instead of taking a walk or getting enough sleep is disrespectful to your well-being. It's time that we started respecting ourselves by taking responsibility for our own health and happiness.

The secret is that there is no secret. No one way works for everyone. You should listen to your own intuition above all else. Everyone wants a quick fix or to believe the hottest new book will have all the answers. But that isn't reality. If you're looking to any one doctor, teacher, writer, trainer, or friend for the answers, then you're not taking responsibility for your own health.

We want to share some useful, reasonable advice to help you reclaim a state of well-being. Wellness is a moving target, meaning it requires constant recalibration and fine-tuning. This is where the "sensible" part of our title comes into play. The life wisdom and good sense you have will help you make critical choices towards well-being. Getting your groove back requires more than eating five servings of vegetables and walking each day. But it isn't nearly as complicated OR time consuming as you think!

Small changes allow us to grow into a new habit and make it a

permanent part of our lives whereas too many sudden changes make it more likely that we revert to old patterns.

So take a lesson from the good old tortoise and just slow it down and let's get into it little by little. Tortoise Power! Change by tiny change, you'll grow healthier, more present, more radiant, and more whole. Following the Four will engender your very best you!

What makes us qualified to dispense wellness advice? We live a healthy, balanced life in the middle of Kentucky, a state that doesn't prioritize health. What's the first thing you think of when you think of Kentucky? Unless you live here, chances are you answered, "Kentucky Fried Chicken," right? Nothing says "health" like a bucket of fried chicken, biscuits, macaroni and cheese, and 32 ounces of tea so sweet it hurts your teeth.

Have you ever seen FX's Justified? Timothy Olyphant plays a US marshal who returns to his home state and ends up battling criminals, meth heads, and religious zealots. It's set in Harlan, just a short drive from us. This is the birthplace of the Hatfields and McCoys, moonshine, snake handlers, and cock fighting.

We hail from a place that doesn't encourage preventive medicine but instead uses its tax dollars to fund programs that deal with the aftermath of poor choices. The common practice here is just too much - too much junk food, too much alcohol, too much smoking, too much TV, too much sitting, too many drugs.

According to the United Health Foundation, Kentucky ranks a lowly 47th in the list of the nation's healthiest states. 29% of Kentuckians smoke and over 33% of us are morbidly obese. In 2013, the New York Times rated the top 100 "hardest places to live in America" based on factors including higher education, median household income, unemployment rate, disability rate, life expectancy, and obesity. The top 6 counties were all in Kentucky!

And yet we wouldn't live anywhere else. Start trash talking Kentucky and we'll put our fighting boots on! Kentucky is one of the most beautiful places on earth with the kindest, most hospitable people you will ever find. This is a place where houses have porches, people love you simply because they know "your people" (by which, they mean your parents, grandparents, uncles, aunts, or cousins, no matter how far removed), and love is generally shown through huge family meals. A place where "y'all" is an actual word.

Rock climbers come from all over the world to climb in our Red River Gorge Nature Preserve. We are home to Mammoth Cave National Park, 38 state parks, 465 lakes, and amazing hiking trails. We believe in bourbon, bluegrass music, basketball, and horse racing. This is a place where the soil will grow most anything and the sunrises and sunsets can soften the hardest heart.

This is our home. And we choose to believe that wellness is the birthright of every person and that it's possible for all. And that starts with first choosing wellness and then educating yourself. You'll have to figure out for yourself how to make it work where you live. If we can do it, anyone can. Here's how.

THE FOUR TO FOLLOW:

INVITE
DIGEST
MOVE
REST

Contents

The Guidelines. Follow the Four!

Invite

Each day, spend five minutes doing one of the following:

Digest

As much as possible:

Move

Each week, try to perform each of these four activities once.

1. Yoga pg 129
2. Resistance Training pg 174
3. Woggle or Walk pg 193
4. Some Movement You Love pg 205

Rest

Every week, engage the rest and digest system in these four ways.

1. Deep Sleep pg 211
2. Restorative Yoga pg 219
3. Self-Care pg 234
4. Nurturing Your Social Connections pg 242

Let's face it; these four things are not hard. Anyone can do this!

1. **INVITE** – Take some time to figure yourself out. Take a personality test, think about what makes you happy, or open your ears to the universe. Just figure out what makes you, you. Invite into your life that which makes you happy and ditch the rest. It's really that simple. Learn to say the word no (nicely, but with intention). Reduce the number of committees, groups, boards or other obligations and simplify to the ones that mean the most to you. If it's volunteering at your kid's school that's got you feeling crazy, figure out a way to contribute that works for you and say no to the rest. Let it go by knowing you are doing your part and that is nothing else is required. Do what you have to do and carve out the other time you have to feed your soul. For your free time, don't over-commit yourself to things that aren't giving you what you need.

2. **DIGEST** – This is simple and no one says it better than our hero, Michael Pollan. "Eat real food, not too much, mostly plants." (Yes, we worship at the Church of Pollan!) We're both librarians and believe that the answer to all of life's problems can be found in a book. But it always seems to come back to Michael Pollan because he consistently makes the most sense out of complicated nutrition. He has become a litmus test for us in that we often say, "what would Michael Pollan say?" He is undoubtedly the most influential food and nutrition writer we have encountered and has significantly influenced our own views as well as this book. He brings the simplicity and pleasure in food back for us, reminding us to eat real food in moderation and enjoy the prep and family time involved in eating.

3. **MOVE** – Your body wants to move. Listen to it! Figure out what movement you like to do and simply do it. Be mindful and think of your body in its current state and not the high school athlete you were 20 years ago. Just like the nutrition world, there are myriad fads and copious amounts of misinformation in the exercise world so start slow and realistic with a view

of the long term. We don't have all the answers but we do know what works for us after many years of trial and error. In fact, boiling our belief down in Michael Pollan language would go something like this: move your body, in different ways, most days.

4. **REST** – Listen to your body and mind. Rest them when they need it. Learn to pay attention to your body's signs of exhaustion. Are your eyes tired? Are you struggling to focus on the task at hand? Take a break and a rest. If this isn't possible, then vow to put yourself in a quiet, dark room early and enjoy a good night's sleep! Andra has to read quietly before falling asleep because it clears her head and allows her to transition to restful sleep. Otherwise, her brain doesn't quite shut off and she lies there thinking about all the things she should have done differently 20 years ago. Talk about unproductive! Take the time to learn what works for you and put those systems in place to achieve the rest your body and mind needs.

PART ONE
INVITE

The thing always happens that you really believe in, and the belief in a thing makes it happen. ~Frank Lloyd Wright

The Roadblocks to Wellness

When asked how we feel on any given day, many of us would too often answer "busy" or "tired". The major roadblocks to wellness are, for most women, time and energy. We'd happily take care of ourselves...if we only had the time!

The thing is, however, that we do have the time. We've just forgotten how to use our time intelligently. We're going to show you how to recapture your energy. In this way, you'll add minutes to the clock.

We often think of our grandparents. Families were much bigger in those days and our grandmothers would have to tend to a garden, cook meals from scratch, clean the house, sew up torn clothes, stay on top of mountains of laundry, stay in touch with far-away relatives with handwritten letters, and somehow maintain their sanity. They had no dishwasher, washing machine, dryer, computer, or cell phone to call Papa John's for dinner. They didn't even own a TV until the early 1960s, which didn't matter since nothing but the test pattern came on until after 3:00 pm.

In comparison, we've got it pretty easy. Technologies like email, texting and the brilliance that is the DVR allow us to do things at lightning speed. We don't have to wait for the mail when we can call our friends pronto. We don't even have to wait until next week to see the next episode of The Walking Dead, but can instead download it online. Amazon delivers our clothes and books and even our toiletries. The grocery store is a cornucopia of convenience foods, from bags of salad to cut fruit. So if we have so much more time to do things previous generations never dreamed possible, why do we feel there is never enough time? Do we really have more real work in our lives than our grandmothers?

We think not. We think the world has gotten really bad at being still. We have gotten addicted to busyness. If we have any free minute, be it waiting in line at the grocery, in the school pick-up line, even at a stoplight, we're texting, emailing, or "working" social media. And we know that it's not just us.

A 2014 study at Harvard showed people left alone in a room for 15 minutes chose mundane tasks over sitting in silent contemplation. They even "preferred to administer electric shocks to themselves instead of being left alone with their thoughts. Most people seem to prefer to be doing something rather than nothing, even if that something is negative". Yikes!

All of this constant busyness fries our brains. Neuroscientists call this "cognitive overload" and since the invention of computers and smart phones, it has gotten much worse. It isn't really that we have less time than our grandparents but that we fill the space with too much crazy and not enough stillness.

Stillness recharges our batteries. If we're willing to spend a few minutes each day getting still, we are much more efficient when it comes to checking things off our to-do list. In this way, if we devote five minutes every morning towards mindfulness, there is a lot less waste in our haste. A lot less haste in every way.

When...Then: Stop Making Excuses

If there are two words that cause us to go to pieces, they are "when…then" used in the same thought. As in, "when I have more time, then I will start walking. When I get the promotion, then I can afford yoga classes. When the kids go to college, then I will meditate." "When…then" is just a veiled excuse. What you really mean is "I'm too busy, too poor, too tired, too apathetic." "When…then" prevents you from living out loud. Your future rests solely in your hands and your willingness to take action.

Whatever excuses you have been making, stop right now. You only have to make one change at a time, but make it already! Can't afford yoga classes? Borrow a DVD from your public library. No time to meditate? Sit in the bathroom stall for a few extra minutes and breathe. If you want peace, that's definitely the place to go! Draw up the blueprint to make the rest of your life the best of your life.

What steps will it take to live your truth? It's going to feel uncomfortable at times. You're going to get frustrated. You'll have days when you wonder if it's all worth it. On those days, spend some time with your vision board and revisit your Why (we'll discuss the what, how, and why of a vision board later on). Lao Tzo famously said, "the journey of a thousand miles starts with one step." Now Lao Tzu strikes me as a guy who takes responsibility for his life as opposed to making excuses for his regrets.

Turn your can'ts into cans and your dreams into plans

The Sanskrit word asana means "seat" and refers to the traditional seated pose where your legs look like a pretzel. Sitting to meditate? Awesome. Sitting because you're too scared or lazy to take charge of your own amazing life? Unacceptable. Now get off your asana and take that first step.

The Practice

Each day, we would encourage you to spend five minutes doing one of the following:

1. Meditation

2. A Breathing Exercise
3. Journaling
4. Gratitude Attitude Training

We'll explain each one in depth and why it can help you find more joy, energy, and presence in your life. But first, we'd love for you to understand the Law of Attraction.

The Universal Law of Attraction

Your imagination is a preview of life's coming attractions.
~Albert Einstein

Intentions drive your actions, either consciously or unconsciously. We're going to show you how to clearly define the life you want.

The idea that our thoughts create our reality comes from physics. Let us explain.

In his Theory of Relativity, Albert Einstein stated that e=mc2. The e in the equation stands for energy. The mc squared stands for a really huge number signifying 99.9% of everything in the cosmos.

Energy = Everything

Most of that everything (like people, plants, stars, walls, mugs, truly everything) is made up of atoms. The atoms that make us up are the same atoms that make up everything else in the universe. As Carl Sagan understood, "the nitrogen in our DNA, the calcium in our teeth, the iron in our blood, the carbon in our apple pies were made in the interiors of collapsing stars. We are made of star stuff." These atoms that compromise everything are constantly moving, like Erin after too much coffee. Sometimes they move slowly and sometimes they move quickly. Even things that are seemingly still - like a wall or a lampshade - are actually moving very, very slowly at a subatomic level. Still with us?

All of this subtle energy is vibrating. This vibratory output creates a measurable frequency. EVERYTHING in the universe is comprised of energy that continuously emits a frequency.

And this brings us to a universal rule called the Law of Attraction. The Law of Attraction states that atoms, and everything they make up, are attracted toward each other to the degree of common use. The Law of Attraction is universal and applies to all the planes of life including physical, emotional, intellectual, and spiritual.

What does this have to do with creating your most radiant life? You attract the things with which you are in vibrational harmony. A positive mental attitude attracts positive experiences while a negative mental attitude attracts negative experiences.

If you're going to change your life, you must start by changing your thoughts.

We all know that person who is constantly negative or unhappy. No matter what happens, they will put a negative spin on it. Their body demonstrates this and they seem to have more than their share of life's misfortunes. We call these people Energy Vampires. Have you noticed when you are around them how they steal your energy? You leave them feeling exhausted and negative yourself. They are actually toxic to your well-being.

Sadness, grief, resentment and fear are low-frequency emotions. Picture your body under the influence of these emotions. The body is listless, the shoulders rolled forward, the eyes cast downward.

We also all know a really happy, positive person. When they're faced with challenges, they handle them with optimism and grace. These are easy people to be around and we feel drawn to them because they lift us up.

Happiness, love, creativity, compassion, and especially gratitude are high-frequency emotions. Now picture your body under the influence of these emotions. The body is energetic, the heart open, the eyes bright. When we choose thoughts that resonate with our highest needs, we are literally inviting those experiences into our life.

It is actually possible to control our genes by controlling our thoughts. It's long been believed that we are victims of our genes and that we have no control over our body functions. But epigenetics is starting to paint a different picture over time. The field of epigenetics refers to the science that studies how the development, functioning and evolution of living things are influenced by forces operating outside the DNA sequence, including environmental and energetic influences (like where we live, what we eat, how we exercise, where our passions and hobbies lie, how much sex we have, and most importantly, what we think).

A 2002 study looked at surgery for patients with debilitating knee pain. The patients were divided into three groups. The surgeons shaved the damaged cartilage in the knee of one group, and flushed the knee joint in another, removing all of the inflammatory material. Both of these processes are standard surgeries for arthritic knees. In the third group, the patients were sedated and told that they had surgery, when in fact they had nothing done to their knee. For the patients not really receiving the surgery, the doctors made the incisions and splashed salt water on the knee as they would in normal surgery. They then sewed up the incisions so it looked like a knee that actually had surgery.

All three groups went through the same physical therapy process and the results were astonishing. The placebo group improved just as much as the other two groups who had surgery. Their knee pain was drastically reduced because they believed the "surgery" went well!

The Law of Attraction, when applied to meditation, breathing exercises, journaling, and "to-do" lists, will help you draw more focus, peace, and mindfulness into your life.

When you choose to lead a mindful, present life, the universe will support your efforts.

Make a Vision Board

Creating vision boards is a fun and easy way to get creative with your dreams. It's powerful to surround yourself with images and positive words to help you stay aligned with your goals and keep your attention on your intention.

You can't claim it if you don't name it!

Vision boards are potent reminders of what our values and priorities are. This exercise is a one-and-done to help you really figure out your priorities.

Before starting this journey, you should be very clear on exactly what your intention is. It's easier to rise to a challenge when you understand exactly why you want to reach those goals. What is your Why? Our Why is quite simple. We want to be around a long time for our children and husbands. We want to get older and not have any health problems. We want to age gracefully and not be on tons of medications. We want to get older and just feel good about ourselves. Yep, that's all there is to it.

To find your Why, ask yourself why you started this journey. What led you to reading these very words at this exact moment in your life? Does high cholesterol run in your family? Do you want to feel more energy to keep up with your children? Do you feel like a sleepwalker in your own life and long to be more present and feel more joy? If your Why is large enough, the How will take care of itself. Let your vision board reveal your Why (and your mantra).

For instance, you may be thinking, "I want to be happier". OK, great start! But what exactly does your particular happy look like? Erin's happy vision would entail spending more time with her family at the beach, a hammock, red wine, tons of unread books, and long afternoons playing her guitar. Andra's conception of joy would also be with her family and with unread books, but she would be baking, camping, hiking, and enjoying a craft beer by the campfire. You need to get very specific when you're talking to the Universe!

How to Make a Vision Board

1. Gather your materials. You'll need some heavy stock paper or poster board, scissors, a glue stick, and a few magazines from which you can cut images and quotes. We love Oprah, Better Homes & Garden, Real Simple, and Yoga Journal for our vision boards. You can use postcards, quotes, photographs - the sky's the limit! We're adding a few pages in this book if you want to test-drive the vision board here. Then you'll always have a copy of your Sensible Wellness Vision Board!

2. Set the mood. You can vision alone or make it a date with your family or girlfriends. We like to pour a glass of wine and find enough room to really spread out.

3. Flip through the magazines and tear out pages with images or words that resonate with you. It's fine if you don't even exact-

ly understand why you are called to a certain picture or quote. The Universe may be whispering something you cannot hear yet.

4. Go through the images and words and begin to lay your favorites on the paper or poster board. Eliminate any images that no longer feel right. Trust your instincts! Don't glue anything down until the board feels "right."

5. Hang your vision board where you can see it every day.

6. You can make another vision board anytime you'd like. We generally make a few every year. Erin has vision boards dating back to high school and while Andra has only recently adopted the vision board, she is a big believer!

Now back to the plan!

1

Meditation

Let's talk about using meditation as medication. Meditation allows us to live a more present, mindful life. It trains the brain to tolerate stressful events and to tone down the body's physical response to those stressors (like a racing heart, a bloodstream flooded with cortisol, sweaty palms, etc.) Meditators have lower blood pressure and cholesterol levels but higher alpha rhythm brain waves (which indicates a calm, relaxed mind).

Think about your route to work. How many times have you traversed it? Do you find that sometimes you arrive at work and can't even remember getting there? The route is deeply ingrained in your brain - it becomes effortless on your part. This is called a neural pathway.

Every time your mind feels anxious or depressed, you're digging a neural trench that makes it easier and easier to feel anxiety or depression in every future situation. The trench becomes your default setting. Mindfulness training builds new paths towards gratitude, kindness, and hope.

With over 80 billion neurons constantly firing, our brains benefit immeasurably from relaxation. Mindfulness training is like a gym membership for your gray matter. Researchers have found that the cerebral cortex (the part of the brain that controls rational thought, language, and emotion) is thicker in meditators than in people who shun meditation.

Myth: I have too many thoughts to meditate well.

Truth: We all have too many thoughts. It's sort of the whole reason people started to meditate! You won't stop thinking when you mediate. But you will start to become more aware of your thought patterns, which makes it easier to change the ones that could use some attention. Some scientists believe that we have between 50,000-70,000 thoughts a day! Meditation will, over time, lengthen the little space between all those thoughts. This means you'll be more responsive and less reactive in your daily life. Our minds always seem to be doing but mindfulness is about being. Meditation is a clear choice to be still and often goes against the "go, go, go" mentality our culture celebrates.

Insu-what?

The insula is a part of your brain deep in the cerebral cortex. Daniel Siegel calls the insula the "the information superhighway" because it connects the cerebral cortex to the rest of the body and all of its sensations. When we meditate regularly, we are actually building new neural pathways in the brain and enlarging our insula. The more mindful we are, the larger our insula and the more we can perceive small sensations. In this way, an apple tastes sweeter or a cashmere sweater feels softer. Over time, we can experience life more intensely and are more easily satisfied. A Dartmouth study found that women with larger insula have more intense orgasms. Now there's a reason to sit your booty down on the meditation cushion!

Meditation helps us harness the power of our thoughts. It helps us focus on what we truly want with clarity and conviction. Remember the Universal Law of Attraction?

Wand Words

Erin's daughter Izzie wants a magic wand for her birthday this year. A magic wand is unique to each individual wizard, providing protection against malevolent forces and lighting the way when it's dark. When used correctly, it's a powerful ally.

For those of us without actual wands, we can use the power of affirmations, namely messages that we would like to ingrain in our lives. Affirmations are carefully chosen words that, when repeated, act as magic wands of light and protection. Think of them as wand words. Words, spoken or thought, produce an actual physical vibration. When we repeat words over and over, the words can have a direct impact on the situation produced.

Affirmations work via the law of attraction. What we think about, we bring about. We have the power to repel or cultivate our dreams. Source is always trying to nurture our success.

How does it work? Repeat the affirmation each morning during your meditation practice, one word per exhale. You can make it work faster by also saying a few rounds throughout the day or before bed. Write your wand word on sticky notes and place them where you'll see them: your fridge, your car, your workspace, wherever they'll fit!

Practice saying your word aloud as you look in the mirror. Say it like you mean it, even striking a power pose or waving an imaginary wand if it helps. Say it as if you're casting a spell (think about how you'd say abracadabra! and you've got the general picture). Just like a guitarist playing scales over and over or a basketball player practicing free throws for hours on end, the more we train our minds to think positively, the deeper we carve a neural pathway to invite more positive things into our lives. The repetition reinforces the power of the wand word.

Want your own wand word? Here are a few to consider. Circle any that resonate with you, and then listen closely to Source over the next few weeks to see which ones keep popping back up in your life. That's your word for now. Give yourself permission to change your wand word as often as needed.

Acceptance, Awareness, Badassery, Balance, Challenge, Connection, Flow, Grace, Gratitude, Intuition, Love, Openness, Peace, Release, Source, Stillness, Trust, Wealth, Wholeness, Wonder.

> **Journal Prompt**: Nothing reinforces your belief in affirmation like verification that it's working. Throughout your affirmation practice, keep a list of all the ways, both big and small, that the Universe is supporting your affirmation. Remember that even mistakes or conflict can be profound lessons in the progress of personal evolution. Be open to the experience!

Before we discuss how to meditate, let's clear up a common misunderstanding about meditation. Meditation is not a religious practice, though it can certainly be a spiritual experience. It won't conflict with your prayers but instead will make the experience of prayer richer. Wiser men than us have described prayer as when we talk to God and meditation as when we listen to God. Having a teacher help you get started is useful, but not necessary. You can buy podcasts and smart phone apps that will walk you through guided meditations if you prefer. You can also go to www.theOMplace.net to access a video of a meditation led by Erin. But we'll also walk you through how to do it at home.

Here's What to Do

Find a comfortable seat, sitting with a tall spine. Roll your shoulders and stretch your neck a bit. Then let your spine sway around a little until you find a really happy place of ease. If you lie down, there's a good chance you'll drift off. Sleep is great, but not the goal of your meditation practice. We are looking for a relaxed awareness. In other words, you'll be really present and calm, but totally aware of that feeling. Relax your shoulders and face. Seal the lips but loosen the jaw so you aren't grinding your teeth. Breathing in and out of your nose, start to observe the rise and fall of your breath. When the breaths feel relaxed, start to repeat your wand word silently on each exhale.

When your mind wanders off, don't engage, attach to, or resist those thoughts. This gives those thoughts the power they need to run amok. Instead, just notice that the mind has wandered off and come back to repeating your wand word.

Your mind will wander off a lot. That's OK! Be gentle and compassionate with yourself. When you notice you're planning, remembering, or worrying, just let those thoughts go and come back to repeating your wand word. Practice for about 3-5 minutes to start, and then slowly add time, as you feel able.

Myth: You don't have time to meditate.

Truth: Every single person in the world has a few minutes each day to sit still and observe their thoughts. I'm pretty sure Oprah is busier than I am, but she finds time to meditate every day. Ditto for Ellen DeGeneres and Arianna Huffington. Even a few minutes of deep, relaxed breathing while sitting still lowers blood pressure and slows heart rate. MRIs taken after short meditation sessions show a decrease in beta waves (which means your brain is processing information) and an increase in alpha waves (which means you're getting into that awesome "flow" state of relaxed awareness). Start with 3 minutes a day and work up to a length that fits your life.

Let's say you're practicing your wand word when you suddenly think, "today is Wednesday." Then notice how the mind makes these wild associative jumps like, "on Wednesdays I meet Sarah at the coffee shop. They have those cute shirts at that coffee shop. What should I wear today? Yesterday I wore heels and my feet hurt. I need a pedicure. At my last pedicure, I ran into Ellen. Did Ellen ever divorce that jerk, Mark? Mark works at the bank. I need to go to the bank tomorrow. The bank is near the dry cleaners, so...."

And on and on it goes. This is called associative thinking and our brains are hardwired to do it. Neurobiologists suggest that the mind wanders away from the present moment 6 to 8 times every minute! The goal isn't to lose your focus. The goal is to notice when you think, "today is Wednesday" and gently return to your wand word. We like to think of all those connected thoughts as cars on a train. Then we mentally choose to stand on the platform and watch the train go by without climbing aboard.

Andra's Addition:

Is This Enlightenment? It Feels like Constipation!

Erin is a truly unique and amazing person. She seems to function on a different frequency than most people. I think of her as this spinning, vibrating little energy sprite, always up early and getting unimaginable amounts of things accomplished before I have even savored my first sip of coffee. She's enviably organized, efficient and focused on whatever she is working on. All of her yoga students, clients, friends and family know that absolutely nothing is done half-assed!

Aside from being intelligent, Erin is continually self-educating and improving her knowledge base. She has a nasty Audible and Amazon habit! She is extremely interesting, vibrant and entertaining to spend time and converse with. She's a great sounding board and we have solved many of life's problems just "talking it out" while walking near our homes on Quisenberry Lane.

Most importantly, she doesn't expect anyone to be like her in any way and truly seems to exist knowing she is the way she is and you are the way you are. Period. I think this acceptance is a result of many years of practicing yoga and meditation but from wherever it comes, it's liberating because she accepts you for just being you.

As we are very close, I have watched, admired and benefited from these qualities in Erin for many years. Truth be told, I have often envied these characteristics, wishing I had just a little here or there. I have come to understand that the main difference between us is simply confidence.

Erin approaches everything with a huge amount of confidence. I struggle with this and am quick to second-guess my abilities with that little voice inside me sometimes saying "are you crazy? You can't do that? Who do you think you are?" As I have aged, that voice has quieted but is still there, lurking in the background. Erin makes many things in this book seem easy, but they are not easy for everyone.

Take meditation, for example. I have always struggled with meditation because I felt it was a waste of precious time that I needed to get my shit done! My expectations were that my body (legs folded in perfect lotus) would levitate off my cushion and I would experience unspeakable and orgasmic enlightenment! This would then solve all the mysteries I've ever tried to solve, while allowing me to finally achieve inner harmony, and literally glide through the rest of my day among mere mortals.

So every time that didn't happen, I was naturally disappointed and frustrated, thus labeling meditation as a colossal waste of time and energy. But then one day, I decided to become a yoga teacher and enrolled myself in the program located literally next to my house (I know, pretty fortunate, right?). I had watched these would-be yoga students come and go for years and it never occurred to me that I might join their ranks one day. But as Darius Rucker so eloquently says in his song, *This*:

All the doors that I had to close
All the things I knew but I didn't know
Thank God for all I missed
Cause it led me here to This

Sing it, Darius! I don't know why or how, but I arrived via this crooked path to become a yoga teacher and personal trainer in my middle 40s. I had completed several personal training contracts and decided to make myself into the kind of personal trainer that I would pay for if I were the customer. My kids were getting older and I needed to find a productive and contributory path for myself as they began to need me less. So, I bopped myself down to yoga teacher training at the OM place excited and eager, albeit a little nervous to find that I was surrounded by a diverse and interesting group of strangers who also wanted to teach yoga to others.

From the beginning, Erin explained that one of our requirements for completion was to begin a daily meditation practice of our own. I saw absolutely no point in such a thing but, having no choice in the matter, I started trying to meditate daily. And by try, I would scrunch my eyes together and strain to hear Source whispering to me in my vain search for "enlightenment." I can tell you that I looked and felt more like I was experiencing constipation than enlightenment!

I despised it at first. But two things began to happen. First, in yoga teacher training, we actually talked about meditation and my understanding began to become much more realistic. Nobody was experiencing levitation - they were just carving out a small bit of quiet time in their busy lives. Second, meditation was different for everyone in my training. This idea that meditation was completely personal had never crossed my mind before. Some people said it worked for them first thing in the morning, others in the car while driving or for some while they were in the bathtub! The thought that you could meditate almost anywhere was crazy and amazing to me.

In the end, I learned that meditation wasn't about mysticism but was simply about being quiet for an amount of time determined by you. Our world is chaotic and busy but even a few minutes of quiet and stillness each day can completely change your outlook. I learned that my meditation time is early in the morning while the house is quiet, clasping my mug of steaming delicious coffee. I just sit still and breathe while thinking about what's in store for me that day. Sometimes I just count my blessings and occasionally I ponder a particular problem I am experiencing.

And you know what I've come to realize? Nothing mystical happens. Let me repeat that - nothing mystical happens! And I am now OK with that and not disappointed in the least. In fact, I don't even expect it, but I definitely find that my day goes better on those mornings that I am still, even for just a little while. I don't try to figure out why this is but breathing in the delicious coffee aroma cleanses my busy mind and sets the course for how I am going to approach my day.

2

Breathing Exercises

You can live over 50 days without food and about a week without water, but without oxygen, the old bod gives out in less than 5 minutes! Breathing is so important and we really should learn to do it correctly. Enter pranayama, the science of breath control. Pra means "always" and na means "moving". The Yogis realized the importance of an adequate oxygen supply thousands of years ago. They developed and perfected various breathing techniques that can help to revitalize the mind and the body. These techniques bring more oxygen to the blood and brain while controlling our life energy.

Breathing supplies our bodies with oxygen while ridding us of waste products and toxins. Oxygen is essential for the proper and efficient functioning of the brain, nerves, glands and other internal organs.

Myth: I don't need to think about how I'm breathing.

Truth: Just because we breathe involuntarily doesn't mean we're breathing efficiently. An average American female has enough lung tissue to cover a tennis court! But most of us only use a fraction of our lung capacity. Poor posture, long-term stress, and environmental toxins mean far too many of us breathe high in the chest, where we take in about a pint of air with each inhale. Learning to breathe in our bellies means we can take in up to a gallon of air with each breath! Watch a baby or a dog breathe; they breathe with their entire bodies. We need to re-learn this skill. Shallow chest breathing means we aren't ridding the body fully of carbon dioxide, which keeps toxins and wastes in our blood stream. Chest breathing does not fully utilize the diaphragm or the larger, lower part of our lungs. Learn to breathe in your belly and improve both the volume of oxygen coming in and the volume of carbon dioxide going out. You will be amazed at how much better you feel.

We breathe about 25,000 times a day through almost 1,500 miles of airways. We all know how to breathe - it happens automatically. So it seems foolish to think that one can be told how to breathe. Yet, one's breathing becomes modified and restricted in various ways through force of habit. We develop unhealthy habits without being aware of it. We use poor posture, resulting in shallow breaths and a diminished lung capacity. We inhale toxins such as smog or cigarette smoke in our environment. We work at high-stress jobs. The more stressed out we are, the tenser our muscles become. This leads to the contraction of the muscles in your arms, neck and chest. The muscles that move the thorax and control inhalation and muscular tenseness clamp down and restrict the exhalation. The breaths become shorter and shorter. After an extended period of intense focusing, the whole system seems to be frozen in a certain posture. We become fatigued from the decreased circulation of blood and from the decreased availability of oxygen for the blood.

Erin's Edition:

Mind the Gap

When I lived in England, I took the tube everywhere. When you board the train, an intercom will remind you to "mind the gap," which is just a charming English way of saying, "Hey idiot! Try to not fall into the hole between the platform and the train!" A mindful life encourages exactly the opposite. When we sit still and become aware of the breath, we notice that there is both an inhale and an exhale. Pay closer attention, and you'll see there is also a tiny pause at the top and bottom of each inhale and exhale too. You don't have to force this little pause to happen - it's already there! You just probably haven't ever noticed it before.

Once you become aware of this gap, you'll see how quiet and peaceful it is there. And this oasis of calm is always available to you. You don't have to lose weight to find it. You don't need an advanced degree to notice it. You simply have to pay attention. Falling into this gap between each breath will lengthen the gap between thoughts in your mind. And in this mind gap, some pretty freaking cool stuff happens!

Have you ever been going about your day, maybe pouring milk over cereal or riffling through the mail, when you get a twinkling that the moment is bigger and more important than it first seems? There is a profound shift of awareness. Your body might buzz a bit and the moment might seem hyper-realistic, like you had just slipped on a pair of glasses and your vision adjusted to High Definition. Sometimes it shows up as déjà vu. Sometimes you feel like Life has hit some metaphysical pause button and time slows way down or stops completely. That is Source awakening in you. Divinity lives inside of you, but you'll only notice it in the gap. When you meditate consistently, you cannot help but awaken to all the miracles around you every day.

When you start looking for the gap, you'll notice this sacred pause exists everywhere. It's the pause in music, with an anticipation of the next note to come. It's the tiny moment at the highest arc of the swing, where you are suspended, transcending the laws of gravity. It's the stop sign, reminding us to stop and pay attention. It's the church bell, prompting us to take heed of passing time and that we have a choice in how we spend that time. It's the rising or setting sun, a baby's laugh, or a short nap. It is in this gap where we learn to respond to our lives, instead of mindlessly reacting all the time. It's our internal reset button.

Now I differentiate between spirituality and religion. You can have divinity without theology. Source may show up to you in the church pew, but She's just as apt to show up as the homeless man panhandling for money. Or as the bird that builds a nest in the tree outside your bedroom window. Or as any moment that arises, however mundane.

I have a complicated and confusing history with religion. I was raised Presbuddhist. My hippie Ram Dass-reading folks practiced transcendental meditation and discussed the Five Precepts of Buddhism at the dinner table, yet still dragged my brother and me to the local Presbyterian Church each Sunday.

The Presbyterians are a fairly open-minded bunch, but the hymns are all dirges written by old, white men and the readings are all too often from the Old Testament, with the Angry God constantly smiting some poor guy over some tiny infraction. It rarely seemed relevant to my angsty, pubescent life.

Presbyterians all but ignore the hot, sexy poetry of Song of Solomon and the violent but interesting end-of-days tale told by Revelations. Plus, I really wanted to be a Methodist, because they had an awesome gym for the youth group and invited cool Christian rock bands to play on Friday nights.

My next-door-neighbor, Karla, went to Catholic School. The nuns interested me greatly, based mostly on my love of the movie The Blues Brothers. Karla laid it out for me. If you talked about menstruation, you went to hell. If you masturbated, you went to hell. If you had sex before you were married, you went to hell. Huh. This didn't jibe with the half-naked Christ with rock-hard abs they had hanging in every classroom, looking for all the world like some divine Chippendales dancer. And that was the end of my interest in Catholicism. I wanted to read about Hell, but not actually go there.

Our other neighbors were Jewish, and that was cool too. They invited us for Passover, where they served exotic dishes while they told stories about what the food meant, prayed in some beautiful foreign language, and let me have tiny sips of wine. But then we were invited to their house for their son's bris. Talk about confusing! No one had prepared me for witnessing a circumcision or the volume of the wail that baby would let out when his foreskin was removed. And that rules out being Jewish too.

When I went to college, I became fascinated with the great philosophers and comparative religion. I discovered Joseph Campbell, Pema Chodron, and Thich Nhat Hanh. I read Thoreau, The Torah, and the Bhagavad Gita. I bellied up to the World Religion buffet and sampled until the zipper broke on my jeans. The more I read about world religions, the more I saw similarities instead of differences. And the more I realized that God had never spoken to me in church.

But I hear Source everywhere these days. Not in a, "Hey Erin, though shall not partake of that extra bread or I shall smite you" kind of way. It's more that, since I started meditating every day, I deepened my sense of awareness and understanding to the point that I can't not see miracles everywhere I look. When you have a consistent stillness practice, you spend more time "in the gap" between thoughts. And as that gap widens, you create space for holiness to arise.

The most spiritual experience of my life happened not in church, but in Nature, where Source is evident everywhere. I was lying on my front porch on an early August morning, an hour or so before the sun rose. I had already meditated and woggled (our unique blend of walking and jogging with just a little booty wiggle) up and down Quisenberry Lane, which primed me to notice the Big Gap about to hit me like a meteor.

I lay on my back to stretch and watch the stars. There was a half moon and the stars looked like Source had poked a million holes in the sky and then turned on a halogen lamp. We don't have street-lights or houses near enough to ruin the moment with light pollution, so it was just me, the interstellar sky, and the crickets singing the one song they know on repeat.

I was just lying there when my body started to buzz and a feeling of mild euphoria and hyper-awareness washed over me. Within the context of this ordinary moment, something extraordinary happened. I felt transcendence flow through me. Rather than making me feel small and insignificant, seeing the far-away galaxies made me feel greater than I was, an absolutely crucial thread in the fabric of the universe.

I know how this sounds, but this was my experience. I felt Divinity course through me. And then I realized I was in the Gap and started thinking my way out of it. Was I hopped up on endorphins from my woggle? Had I had too much coffee? It was at this moment, a falling star streaked across the sky. In actuality, a falling star is a meteoroid that burns up as it falls into Earth's atmosphere, but the term "falling star" is perfectly apt. This celestial light show was clearly Divinity reminding me to stop over-thinking the experience and take it as the miracle it so clearly was.

So I would encourage you to take advantage of these Gaps. Start looking everywhere for Gaps in the world. Look for Gaps in your thoughts, in your breath, in the space between you and what you perceive as solid. Then start noticing how these Gaps create space for moments of holiness in your life. When you take time for the Gap, you'll start mindfully responding to life rather than mindlessly reacting to it. After the Gap, life resumes. But you are so much more present in that life.

> **Journal Prompt**: What connotations does the word "faith" have for you? What were you raised to believe? Do you now reject or embrace those beliefs?

Connecting to Source

Have you ever heard of a Chladni plate? Named for a German musician and physicist, Ernst Chladni is sometimes called "the father of acoustics". Basically, he sprinkled sand on a metal plate and then drew a violin bow across the side of the plate. The sand reacted to various frequencies, shaking themselves into these beautiful patterns. Seriously, set this book down and YouTube Chladni plates right now to watch this incredible vibration dance. We'll wait. Did you do it? Totally awesome, right? You're welcome.

So anyway, those gorgeous sand patterns are now called Chladni figures and are used in the design of wooden acoustic instruments like cellos and guitars. In fact, Erin just bought a beautiful Martin guitar designed in this exact fashion! Our point is that just because we can't see something doesn't mean it isn't exerting a great and powerful force in our lives.

We call this unseeable power Source. You might call it God, Allah, Yahweh, Brahmin, Spirit, Kismet, Nature, The Breath, The Big Kahuna, or The Big Lebowski. Yoda calls it The Force. Liz Gilbert writes about "Big Magic". Nikola Tesla names it simply vibration. We don't care what name you use to describe the unseen powers of the cosmos. But we would strongly encourage you to acknowledge they exist. Having faith in Source will make your wellness journey far easier. Source supplies an infinite amount of cosmic abundance and most of us exist on mere crumbs of awesome. If you want to truly get yours, then belly up to the Source Bar.

Having faith in Source will make your wellness journey far easier. Source reminds us that each individual on the planet totally matters. This is great news for those times when we feel overwhelmed by life and we just want to curl up in a giant bag of potato chips. We have a responsibility to take care of ourselves because we play an important role in Source. But Source also reminds us that we are but a tiny speck of dust on a tiny blue dot in one universe of billions. This necessary perspective keeps us from taking it all too seriously or feeling like our problems are the most important ones ever. But best of all? Source reminds us to let go and trust that it will all be OK. And Source gives us infinite do-overs to relearn this message as many times as it takes.

There are many ways to hear the divine melody of Source. Meditation, prayer, having a gratitude practice, attending church, journaling, eating well, moving your body, practicing yoga, forgiving, being in nature, having sex, spending time with friends, sleeping deeply, laughing, hugging, taking care of others, doing anything that lights your inner fire. Basically, following the four!

Remember the law of attraction? High frequency activities, thoughts, and emotions attract other high frequencies (Source). Honoring invite, digest, move, and rest raises your vibrational frequency and that connects you to Source. A strong tie to a higher power creates more peace, joy, and contentment in your life. It also strengthens your resolve to figure out what things best support your individual path to wellness. A lack of spiritual awareness attracts negativity and poor health. So spend some time clarifying your beliefs surrounding a higher power.

> **Journal Prompt**: To connect more deeply to Source, what changes would you need to make in your life? What would you add or subtract from your life?

Try This Breathing Exercise

Set your smart phone timer for 5 minutes. Sit comfortably and rest your hands on your knees with the palms up. Draw the awareness to the tip of the nose. Notice the breath as it enters and exits the body. Like life itself, it comes and goes. Allow the next inhale to happen and, as you exhale, touch the thumb to the index finger and silently say, "one." Breathe in. Breathe out and touch the thumb to the middle finger and silently say, "two."

Continue in this way without allowing the breath to become too rapid or shallow. If you lose your count, it's no problem. The aim is to focus on the movement and sound of the breath, not to reach a certain number quickly. We like to tell our yoga students "no hurry, no worry." Just start again. When the timer rings, open the eyes and notice how you feel.

3

Journaling

Writing allows us to better understand ourselves and how we fit into the world at large. A journal is an outlet without judgment, ridicule, or blame. The act of writing accesses our left brain, the rational, analytical part. When we keep the left hemisphere of the brain busy through writing, it frees the right brain up to create and discern. In this way, we strengthen our powers of intuition and understanding.

Wondering how to get started? The beauty of journaling is that there are no rules except that what you write is for your eyes only. Buy yourself a lovely journal, something that is beautiful and inviting. It is also a lovely place to keep ticket stubs and photos as you write about those events (the main reason we don't journal electronically). Invest in a really nice pen or set of colored markers. Erin is partial to blue medium point uniball signos, the only pen with which she'll journal.

> *Myth: I have to be a good writer to journal.*
>
> *Truth: When you journal, you're only writing to and for yourself, so it doesn't matter how well you write. Give yourself permission to simply write, with no judgment or shame. In fact, you don't have to write in words at all! You can doodle or draw if that floats your boat. There is no right or wrong way to journal. It is simply a way to*

process your thoughts and experiences.

When you start writing, don't worry about punctuation or grammar. Just write down ideas as they come. Don't sensor your thoughts or try to make yourself appear smarter, kinder, or more insightful. Just be truthful! Try to write for 5-15 minutes. We find it's best to do it at the same time every day - we like to do it first thing in the morning as we drink our coffee. You can doodle, jot down ideas, detail the happenings of the day, ponder the great mysteries of life, or list songs that make you happy. We've written letters to our future selves, transcribed the birth story of our children to give them one day, and composed poems and songs. Make sure to date each entry, as you'll be happy years later if you ever reread your journal (we do all the time)!

> **Journal Prompt**: What is your biggest worry right now? Is it a realistic concern? Is there anything you can do about them? Write about the worst case scenario. If this happens, then I will...

Andra's Addition:

Find Your Write Reasons and Shut Yourself Up

I'm sure it's no surprise that both journaling and writing don't come easy for me. Well, writing comes easy...but writing about myself (which is essentially journaling) does not! I'd rather have a root canal or a really heavy period!

This subtle distinction has been a bit of a shock for me. I'm a librarian for goodness' sake! I love books and words and order. I can almost smell a well-ordered environment because a peace and stillness come over my body and mind. It doesn't even have to be a library - it can be any structured environment. I've even had it happen in our local orthodontics office. It's an absolute machine of efficiency in there and I always love just sitting in the waiting room!

I know it's ridiculous but it's true for me and I have long known and embraced this about myself. Other than loving books and research, order is the third reason I became a librarian. I simply love to be surrounded by order. My mom and dad have always said that as a child, I would arrange my toys rather than play with them. In college, I used to love taking the chaos of writing a research paper and ordering it into a cohesive end product. So naturally I thought writing a book would be easy.

Wrong, wrong and way wrong! Writing a book isn't hard but writing a book that contains my preferences, secrets and emotional knick knacks is absolute torture. "I'd like a little bit more of the juicy personal bits from you, Andra," my editor would say in a delightful Irish accent, as my insides rolled. "OK, more personal stuff. I get it," I would respond with veiled fright.

But at home, I would find a toilet that had to be cleaned right that moment, or a drawer that must be dealt with even though no one has looked in it for 11 years. You get the idea. I would rather write about something or help edit something Erin has written, than put anything down about myself. I think it's the permanence that scares me and makes me feel so vulnerable. I feel like I'm exposing my soul and my secrets for all to see and judge. And that makes me really uncomfortable.

As you know, Erin and I are the closest of friends with an intertwined history and life. But the journey of this book alone has taken us in a different, uncharted direction. Not bad, just different. Erin has always been a writer and journal-filler so this book came unsurprisingly easy for her. During this process, I have often been frustrated at the ease with which she can just openly write about herself. I am much more guarded with my feelings but I have come to realize that this is just who I am whether I like it or not.

As I struggled to write for this book, I would hear that little voice in my head that I have always heard saying, "you can't write a book. Who do you think you are?" or, "this is so stupid. No one is going to read this!" This voice has always been part of my inner dialog as long as I can remember. I think it's just how I'm made, part of my personality. Sometimes I can override it and prove it wrong, but sometimes I give in and let it convince me. The best thing about this voice is that as I get older, I am getting better at silencing it.

When I see stories of the human atrocities happening around the world where people are struggling to live just a normal life, it makes it me feel bad that I so selfishly struggle with this stupid negative voice in my head. I have so much ease and comfort - the least I could do is believe in myself. At the very least I can and should just believe in myself and stop listening to that stupid voice. Why not? What do I really have to lose?

As this writing journey progressed, I began to realize that my inner voice is a critical bitch and she doesn't always tell the truth. Just like the devil on your shoulder that whispers about how fat, or stupid, or old and dried up you are, there is really no place for this voice. You and I have a choice - we don't have to listen to that voice. It may not go away, but we don't have to listen. The voice may rattle on, but we can disregard what it has to say.

When I observe our girls, Connley and Izzie, I don't see the nasty voice present in either of them. Their self-confidence seems to fill every room they inhabit and I truly hope it stays that way. My hope is that I haven't passed this onto them and my wish for them is that their inner voice is not an overly-negative nagging witch, but a supportive, kind, pragmatic encouraging voice that cheerleads, "You can and you should!" Because at the end of it all, we all can and we all most certainly should, no matter what that voice tells us.

4

Gratitude Attitude Practice

One of the easiest ways to enact INVITE in your life is by cultivating an attitude of gratitude. One of the main differences between happy people and unhappy people is their level of gratitude. Gratitude is one of the highest emotional frequencies, an emotion expressing appreciation for what we have (as opposed to what we want). It raises our vibration and connects us to Source.

Having a gratitude practice is an integral component of health and wellness. Learning to say "thank you" can literally change your life.

We must cultivate gratitude practices to strengthen our feelings of blessedness. We need to both acknowledge our blessings and recognize that they come from outside ourselves. It opens our heart when we understand that blessings come from other people, nature, or a higher power.

Erin's Edition:

The Terrible Beauty of Losing Your Shit

Ten years ago, I found out I was pregnant. Since I had been taking birth control pills for 16 years and actively trying not to get pregnant, this came as quite a shock. (Aside to my daughter Izzie: when you read this later, know that though you were unplanned, you were not unwelcome. We were not planning to have kids, but you have turned out to be the greatest joy in my life). But I took to pregnancy like I was born for it.

For 9 months, I was drunk on my own female power. I felt strong and beautiful, like a fertility goddess incarnate. Before, if I had gained weight, it would be a catalyst for body image issues, sending me into a spiral of self-loathing. But when I was carrying Isabelle, I loved the soft curves of my hips and my full breasts. I had that pregnancy glow everyone talks about.

It makes so much sense that a baby grows in its mother's belly. The navel chakra is our energetic center, where our life force radiates. That chakra is the chakra of commitment and every day I would assert my commitment to being the world's greatest mother. I was ready to rock that job like I'd rocked everything else in my life, through sheer determination and an unshakable belief that everything would be OK.

And then she was born. I should have known it would be a rocky road when I was overdue and so swollen I couldn't see my feet. I was due on April 1st but the April Fool's joke was on me as that stubborn little girl didn't make her entrance into the world until ten days later. A nurse handed me this wrinkly, squalling thing and I completely went to pieces. She was weird and loud and I was suddenly certain I would be the worst parent ever. The baby I had been dreaming about for nine months had big blue eyes and blonde curls like me. The baby I was handed resembled a monkey more than an infant, with her gigantic feet, skinny legs, big nose, and dark hair.

Then someone whisked her off to the nursery for some tests and I got to sleep for what felt like six full minutes. I was jarred awake to the sound of screaming in my ear. My first thought was that a truck had driven through my vagina. My second thought was that someone needed to shut that baby up. I then realized it was my baby! I knew in that moment that I had no idea how to shut up my own baby.

I started to cry and the nurse had to attach the baby to my nipple to nurse. By this time I was sobbing louder than the baby. The nurse assured me that it was "just the hormones" and that I would feel better in a few days.

That nurse was a dirty liar. I cried for about six months straight. Looking back, it's clear I had some post-partum depression. But in the moment, I was simply convinced that every woman on the planet possessed some maternal instinct I simply lacked.

I would call Andra and be wailing so emphatically I couldn't speak. She would pick up the phone (this being the day of landlines without caller ID) and hear weeping. It only took a second for her to realize it was me and she would gently talk me down off the ledge.

No, she didn't think Izzie had transient neonatal pustular melanosis, it was probably just dry skin, and hadn't she told me to stop reading medical encyclopedias already? No, she didn't think my baby cried more than other babies, she cried an entirely normal amount. No, she assured me, baby poop comes in all sorts of colors and it wasn't supposed to look like chocolate fro-yo all the time and

I absolutely shouldn't call an ambulance. I was an absolute mess.

Some days it felt like Izzie screamed all day and for no apparent reason. By the time David would return from work, I would be a snotty mess. I finally understood why people sometimes shake their babies. It's horrible, but your nerves just get so frazzled. My hours were filled taking care of an infant, so there was no time for self-care. I remember thinking I would be content to never have sex again.

There was a day when Izzie was about two weeks old that I tried to give her away to the UPS man. She had screamed all day long. My emotions were already fragile from the post-partum hormones, so I was a wreck after listening to her wail for five solid hours. When the UPS man knocked, I answered the door with baby vomit in my hair, milk on my shirt, and snot running down my face. I held her out to him and begged him to take her far, far away. I offered him my car and all the cash in my purse if he would take her. I scared the poor man to death! He didn't know what to say to this hysterical woman, so he just slowly backed away from me, dropping my package as he ran to his truck. For months after, he would leave my packages at the end of our driveway rather than bring them to the door.

When Izzie was 5 months old, the Gulf Coast was hit by Hurricane Katrina. David and I considered New Orleans a sort of home away from home, having spent countless hours in smoky jazz bars in the Quarter and eaten numerous beignets with café au lait.

For days, I watched newscasts of dead bodies floating through city streets, the sick and dying waiting on their roofs for the National Guard. It looked like film of some third world country. 20,000 people flocked to the New Orleans Superdome, where toilets quickly overflowed and the air conditioning broke. A section of the roof was torn off in the hurricane, and water rushed in. There were reports that people were raped and murdered in the mayhem.

This event hit me viscerally in a way 9/11 hadn't, because now I was a mother and understood on the deepest level what these people had lost. I felt ashamed at how much energy I had spent feeling sorry for myself, embarrassed by how many hours I spent resenting my child instead of loving her. I decided it was time to remember my blessings and stop feeling awful all the time.

So that week I picked up my journal and wrote. I sat down and meditated. I laced up my shoes and took walks. I started eating more vegetables and drinking less wine. My first journal entry in months was only one paragraph, my meditation lasted only three minutes and my walk not much longer. And if I told you I gave up wine totally, I'd be a big fat liar. It took a lot of time and effort, but eventually I found my way, tiny step by tiny step, back to Me.

And I cannot tell you how grateful I am for that time. Sometimes we need to have a complete go-to-pieces to appreciate fully getting our shit together. The dark times give us perspective. So if you're in dark days now, and all of this seems insurmountable, take heart. It is possible to regain your balance after falling off the wellness wagon.

I have a sign in the yoga studio that says, "Gratitude or Attitude?" I tell my students when we are meditating that everything that happens to us is part of a bigger plan. In yoga, it's called our dharma, or life path. Some think of it as fate or destiny. The free will part occurs in our response to those experiences, in how we perceive the happenings in our lives.

Do we pull our hair and gnash our teeth and ask, "why me?" Do we feel victimized by life? Or do we see every occurrence as a gift, as an opportunity to grow and learn? Dark days are inevitable in life, but they do not have to be permanent. It's worth remembering that when things feel like they are falling apart, they may simply be falling into place.

An easy way to cultivate gratitude is to simply list several things you are grateful for upon waking each day (or silently list them before you go to sleep). Robert Emmons, is the world's foremost gratitude researcher. His studies suggest that people who keep gratitude lists (both written and spoken) are sick less, attain personal goals more, have deeper and longer sleep, and exhibit a greater sense of feeling connected to others than people who do not. Just like in Judith Viorst's classic book, even on the most terrible, horrible, no-good, very bad days, there are blessings to be found. This is an easy and wonderful way for anybody to cultivate feelings of thankfulness.

We can complain because rose bushes have thorns, or rejoice because thorn bushes have roses. ~Abraham Lincoln

A great way to foster appreciation is by playing *A Rose & A Thorn* each day. Each person present tells a "thorn" that happened that day (something that was challenging, unlucky, stressful, scary, or sad). This validates our feelings by acknowledging that life isn't perfect and bad things sometimes happen. It also leads to discussions about how that person could have reacted or handled the situation more mindfully. Then the person must list at least one "rose" from the day - a moment that was sweet, uplifting, or exhilarating. Identifying both a rose and thorn often shows us that they are both a part of the whole and that the thorn often brings about the rose.

But I Want It to Work Now!

So let's imagine you've been performing an Invite Exercise each day. But your life isn't changing. What's up with that? Remember the Law of Attraction? Repulsion is its antithesis but the best way to think of repulsion is resistance. Once, when Erin was learning to drive, she drove a friend's car halfway down the street with the emergency brake on. The car was moving forward but there was a lot of resistance! If your manifestation has yet to arrive, ask yourself how you are resisting. You have to truly believe that your life will improve!

Negative Self-Talk

We've all done it. Yes, even those of us who are totally gung-ho about body acceptance and positive body image. Negative self-talk refers to any thoughts or words that put you down to yourself or to others.

We are more than our bodies.

But as women, we often act like a beautiful body is the only thing that's to be valued. We silently believe that the best way to bond is by dragging ourselves down. We act as if the world only sees us as a body and only accepts us if we look a certain way.

The Sanskrit word yoga means "to yoke", or to bring together body, mind, and soul. You cannot care for your body without also caring for your mind and soul. Acceptance is an on-going practice and one we want you to adopt.

People who are more positive have a better shot of getting and staying healthy. And gosh knows that living in a more positive headspace just makes your life better. That's why meditation is such an important part of your wellness component. When you are choosing to be present in the moment, you create an acceptance of that moment which allows your focus to expand to what really matters. What matters is a strong, healthy body. Not one that strictly adheres to some pie-in-the-sky notion of beauty or thinness. Comparing ourselves to others is ridiculous.

The oak tree would never compare itself to the weeping willow. They are both beautiful and strong in their own unique ways. Start celebrating your own shining light.

This is one of the reasons we have included journal prompts throughout this book. Journaling is a great way to gain perspective on your thoughts. You may notice when you write just how many negative thoughts you truly have. Noticing them is the first step in replacing them with a more positive outlook.

So let's agree to put the kibosh on negative self-talk. Next time you look in the mirror and a negative thought arises, close your eyes and choose a wand word that emphasizes your complete awesomeness (try beautiful, gorgeous, or – our personal favorite – badass). Because you are.

Erin's Edition:

Set Your Expectations to Lara Bar

I am open to the guidance of synchronicity, and do not let expectations hinder my path. ~Dalai Lama

Last year, I led a yoga retreat to Tulum, Mexico. After snorkeling one day, I announced I was hungry. Andra handed me a Lara Bar.

For those of you who have never eaten one, let me explain. A Lara Bar is a clean, whole-food bar made of unsweetened fruits, nuts and spices. I tried the Peanut Butter Cookie version. The ingredients list peanuts, dates, and sea salt. Minimal processing, real food, I'm in!

I dug in with gusto and literally spat the first bite out and scraped my tongue with my fingernail. Imagine you have a moldy date. Now press a rancid peanut into it, roll it around in your sweaty hands, and then shove it down in your pocket. In a week or so, take it out and eat it. That's what that Lara Bar tasted like. "What the hell?" I glared at Andra as I spat it on the ground. She shrugged nonchalantly. "Don't blame me. Your expectations screwed you."

So a few days later, we're standing in line at the Delta counter, waiting to check our bags for the return flight home. The line was long, the airport was hot, and it had been a long time since breakfast. I may have mentioned that I don't ever go long without food. I was getting pretty hangry.

Twenty minutes later, the line seemingly hadn't moved. I started to panic that we won't have time to eat before we board the plane. My hands started to shake a little - I have really low blood pressure and this is my personal sign that I have about three minutes to get some food into my system before I go bat-shit crazy.

Andra, bless her heart, reached into her bag and handed me Cashew Cookie (only ingredients are dates and cashews). "Set your expectations to Lara Bar," she advised.

Oh, my expectations were set low for sure. But desperate times call for desperate measures. I took the first bite and it wasn't so bad.

By the third bite, I was already perking up. It was great! It saved me from meltdown and probably the sanity of my seatmates on the plane.

How much of the stress, anger, frustration, or pain in our lives comes from unrealistic expectations? In the yoga tradition, there is a term called santosha (literally translated as "contentment"). It means to live your life from a place of complete acceptance. Santosha supposes that inner peace arises from our ability to accept whatever life offers us without judgment. It reminds us that there is no need for our lives to be any different at any moment, that every moment is the perfect moment.

You might accept santosha now while calmly reading this, but know it may be hard for you to accept that every moment is the perfect moment. The next time you are frustrated, disappointed or angry, ask yourself if your expectations are simply too high? Are they unrealistic for the situation and setting you up for disappointment?

"Set your expectations to Lara Bar" is now in the lexicon of both our families. When we say it, we really mean to let go of expectations in general. Ridding yourself of expectations doesn't mean you can't be hopeful. Hope is something we create internally through our dreams, our goals, and our thoughts (what we INVITE into our lives, remember?) Hope does not need others to be involved in our journey.

Expectations are a completely different thing. Willy Shakespeare got it right when he said, "expectation is the root of all heartache." Expectations arise from a place of knee-jerk reaction to the moment, from judgment and control. We want things to be a certain way based on our opinions, beliefs, and experiences. Then, when the reality doesn't match our expectation, we feel anger, sadness, or frustration. We get hung up on "how it's supposed to be" and miss the beauty of "how it is."

How do we let go of expectations to be more present and realistic? I bet you've already answered this one. Meditation (see, you were right)! Expectations are just like all the other thoughts racing around our monkey mind — they arise and pass away on their own. Simply observing them with the knowledge that they are making your path harder helps us let them go. And there is no better place to practice this than on the meditation cushion, where you're observing your thoughts without judgment.

> **Journal Prompt**: Who do I appreciate and in what ways am I fortunate? Write down at least 12 things you're grateful for in this moment.

PART TWO
DIGEST

Each year, Americans spend $260 billion on cosmetics, hair products, and goods that promise to make us look younger. Women spend a lot of money, time, and effort on their outer appearance. Then they will fill this beautiful package with garbage!

If we can more mindfully fill our insides with high quality food, the outside will shine beautifully on its own. We want you to learn to nourish yourself intelligently.

So what in the world is high-quality food? It's literally all around you - you just have to know where to look. Our home is Kentucky, which currently boasts the fifth-highest adult obesity rate in the nation. We rank sixth in the nation for obese toddlers and first in the nation for obese high-school students. We live in a state that prioritizes processed food over real food with over 90% of the purchased grocery products in our state being of the nasty, processed variety. We clearly have a quantity over quality problem as we're eating more, but not eating well.

The town we call home is actually a food desert, a designation given to certain areas of the country by the United States Department of Agriculture where a significant number of low-income residents are more than 1 mile (urban) or 10 miles (rural) from a supermarket. The term has also evolved to consider areas where fast food and chain restaurants far outnumber locally owned restaurants where food is prepared by hand (rather than trucked in and reheated). We understand the struggle to put real, nutrient-rich food on our tables day after day.

Food is something that nourishes us by providing nutrients (a huge deposit in our wellness account). A nutrient is any substance in food that provides energy, helps your body "burn" another nutrient to provide energy, and helps build or repair tissue.

Real food has a short shelf life or spoils if not refrigerated. Real food is pictured on a food pyramid. When was the last time you saw Doritos or gummy bears on a food pyramid?

Processed food is CRAP!
Carbonated beverages
Refined sugar
Artificial colors
Processed products

Food is something that comes FROM a plant; CRAP is something that is made IN a plant.

CRAP foods are anti-nutrients, meaning they require more nutrients to digest than the body gets from them (depleting our wellness account). They are worse than empty calories because they actually strip your body of nutrients. Over time, CRAP creates chronic inflammation in your gut.

There are two types of inflammation in our bodies. One is acute inflammation. For example, if you cut yourself, your immune system sends more white blood cells to the site to heal it. Or if you lift weights one day and the next day you're a little sore. Those muscles are slightly inflamed. You created micro-tears in the muscle fibers and triggered that immune response. That short-lived inflammation helps you build stronger muscles. This is inflammation doing its job!

The other kind of inflammation is chronic inflammation. Chronic inflammation is akin to our bodies rusting from the inside. Just as metal rusts when exposed to oxygen, inflammation is caused when oxygen-rich free radicals attack healthy cells and tissues. When we have a high-stress life, we often put CRAP into our bodies. This irritates the lining of our gut and triggers the immune response.

70-80% of our immune system is stationed in our gut. Basically, when you eat CRAP, your body thinks it's being harmed and sends extra blood to try and remedy the problem. This extra blood then creates inflammation. The problem is that the gut can never heal because you never give it a break from the CRAP. This chronic, low-level inflammation sets you up for all the so-called "lifestyle diseases," not to mention gas, insomnia, acne, and lethargy.

It's time to break the cycle! It's time to learn how to intelligently nourish our bodies. Mother Nature is truly the world's greatest pharmacist. Wouldn't it be nice to let your dinner be your doctor?

We're so blessed to live out in the country. This means, on any given day, we are likely to see not only our dogs and cats, but also bison, cows, horses, chickens, deer, skunks, opossums, turkeys, hawks, squirrels, voles, groundhogs, bats, raccoons, snakes, lizards, spiders, foxes, and coyotes. Some are carnivores, others are herbivores. Some are mammals, others reptiles or birds. Some have fur, others have feathers or scales. What do all of these animals have in common? All of these animals are naturally strong because they eat healthy, real food they find in their environment. They've figured it out. And so have we.

But this knowledge was hard-won. Eating well hasn't come easily or quickly for us. We've been on this journey making mistakes and learning for quite some time and have struggled as much as anybody with calorie-counting and dieting. Just take a look at our nutritional histories.

Andra's Addition:

I struggled with an eating disorder in my twenties. It came from a place of control. After several personal tragedies, I became a vegetarian as a way to deal with my sadness. This arose from my need to feel like something in my life was neat and tidy and the "rules" of being a vegetarian resonated with me. A year in, I noticed how awful I felt all the time. I stopped menstruating and was easily 25 pounds underweight.

After having to sit down in an aerobics class, I decided it was time to make a change. So I ordered a sausage and cheese pizza on the spot and it remains to this day the best pizza I have ever eaten. It reminded me that food was a good thing, not something we should use to punish ourselves. I added back protein and more calories to my diet. When some time had passed and I felt better, I reflected back on that dark time. I realized that moderation was not only the best way to eat, but the best way to live my life as a whole.

Erin's Edition:

I was raised in a family that prided themselves on eating wholesome, nutritious food. My family sat down together to enjoy mostly vegetarian dishes when I was young but by middle school, those dinners were a thing of the past. I was in gymnastics and competitive cheerleading and my mom spent every minute she wasn't working driving her daughter to one practice or another. My brother, Ian, played soccer and my father was the high-school soccer coach. The four of us were never home until way past dark and meals were grabbed on the go at fast food restaurants.

I'd grab a banana on the way out of the house in the morning, eat school lunches of fries and more fries, and scarf an equally awful meal on a break at the gym. I drank caffeinated sodas to keep my tank full all day. I was fit from the movement, but was still 10 pounds overweight and suffered from embarrassing acne. It wasn't until my 30s that I really put all the puzzle pieces of wellness together. Now, in my 40s, I'm stronger and more whole than I ever was in my 20s!

Everyone has struggled with eating well. Everyone has a complicated history with eating. But you're not alone. Whatever your struggle was or is, we've been there. And today is the day that it all changes. Today is the day you learn the basics of nutrition so you can start experimenting with what works for your own body - physically, mentally, and emotionally.

Unlike a diet, eating doesn't have a start and end. Eating is a life-long journey of constant enjoyment and requires a flexible, open mind. Finding out what works for you will take some time. But here's an easy place to start because the rules are pretty simple. We will show you how to replace CRAP with nutrition.

1

Carbonated Beverages

Soda is the devil. It truly is. It's devoid of any nutritional value and leads to obesity and diabetes. Yet soda accounts for a quarter of all drinks consumed in the United States. A single can of soda contains the equivalent of 10 teaspoons of sugar. Diet soda is even worse! Diet drinks often contain aspartame, which has been linked to tons of health problems including brain tumors, diabetes, and multiple sclerosis. If you are a soda drinker, you really and truly need to stop right and vow never to drink them again.

So what should you drink instead? Water, coffee, tea, and (moderate amounts of) alcohol.

Water

Water is an essential element. In fact, it makes up more than 70 percent of your body weight. Among other functions, water moistens tissues, regulates body temperature, cushions joints, helps the body absorb nutrients, and flushes out waste products. You could go weeks without food, but take away the H2O and you'll last only a few days!

Ayurveda suggests you drink your water at room temperature or even slightly warm to aid digestion. Cold water causes the muscles and blood vessels in your gut to constrict. Warm water relaxes those same tissues. We lose up to 10 cups of water each day, so aim to drink more water. How much is enough? If you care to know, at least as many ounces as half your body weight each.

But as champions of common sense, we will suggest a crazy idea. Drink when you are thirsty.

Add some lemon! Warm lemon water promotes peristalsis, the stomach contractions that digest your food. Lemon water also creates an alkalizing powerhouse. We would love for you to adopt the habit of drinking a cup of lemon water first thing each morning. Your body gets dehydrated when you sleep and downing a cup of lemon water right out of the gate sets you up to feel better all day. Erin's father, Rankin, is a dentist and suggests drinking that water through a straw to protect your teeth enamel from the acidic citrus.

And remember that your body doesn't absorb large amounts of water well all at once. It's better to sip throughout the day than down a giant glass in one sitting.

Myth: Water flushes out toxins.

Truth: Your kidneys rid the bloodstream of toxins via urine. Drinking extra water does not help the kidneys do their job. But dehydration will slow down how effectively your kidneys operate. If you drink every time you're thirsty, you're probably drinking plenty of water.

Coco Coffee

Coffee is loaded with antioxidants and beneficial nutrients that can improve your health. There's no better way to start your day than the smell of a hot cup of coffee.

There are plenty of hard-core health nuts out there ready to take us to task for suggesting caffeine and alcohol are healthful. We truly feel that, in moderation, both are. We also truly feel that, for us, a life without coffee, tea, beer, and wine is no life at all. Caffeine has been shown to boost memory and exercise performance. Studies show promise in its use to prevent Alzheimer's disease, something we are more and more concerned with as our parents get older. Other studies suggest it decreases bone density and increases blood pressure. It certainly can prevent you from sleeping well if you're over-imbibing. And caffeine is the most commonly consumed psychoactive substance in the world.

When you drink a cup of coffee, the caffeine is absorbed, via the digestive tract, into the bloodstream and travels into the brain. Here, it blocks adenosine, a neurotransmitter that can make you sleepy. Have you ever wondered how your cat can fall asleep in seconds? Adenosine levels increase continuously in cat brains when they are awake, until their brains basically shut down and force them to sleep so adenosine levels can drop again. When humans inhibit this sleepy neurotransmitter by drinking coffee, we feel alert and focused. Another neurotransmitter called dopamine increases, leading to feelings of mild euphoria. So we want to drink more, chasing the focused high.

So we say have your coffee, in moderation. Add value to that "cup of joe" by making it Coco Coffee. No, not cocoa coffee! That does sound delicious, but starting your day with a cup of sugar-laced java is not the way to get going! It may give you a quick burst, but that'll be followed by a sugar crash. We're talking about Coco Coffee, which is simply adding a tablespoon of coconut oil to your coffee.

Sounds disgusting, right? Like it would be greasy and foul? We promise it isn't! Refined coconut oil is very different from most other cooking oils and contains a unique composition of fatty acids. These fatty acids go straight from the digestive tract to the liver, where they are able to provide a quick source of energy.

Tea

We adore tea. Hot, cold, caffeinated, caffeine-free, with honey, with lemon, even with bourbon every now and then. Tea comes from the *camellia sinensis* plant and includes four varieties: green, black, white, and oolong. All of those other "herb" teas are really just infusions of dried plants other than *camellia sinensis*. But both kinds contain an abundance of an antioxidant called polyphenols. Polyphenols protect cells and body chemicals against damage caused by free radicals, which can damage DNA in the body. Numerous studies suggest drinking tea protects against all kinds of cancer.

Erin's Edition:

I traveled all over Central and South America when I was younger, where my passion for coffee was fostered. Even in places where it wasn't safe to drink the water, you could often safely order coffee, since it was boiled in the process. I first remember drinking coffee when I was 6 and in Guatamala. It was a little bitter and pungent to my palate, but I felt grown up sipping a mug of hot coffee with my folks, so I just dumped a half cup of sugar in there and before long I was addicted.

It wasn't until sophomore year of college that I developed a taste for tea. Tea, in my part of the world, is sweet. And by sweet, I mean syrupy sweet. In the South, tea ain't tea unless it tastes like a liquid dessert. And sugar wasn't ever my dietary demon.

In 1992, I lived in London as part of my college's study abroad program. England isn't a country known for its fabulous coffee. Tea is not only king here, it is an experience. Every day around 4:00 pm, pretty much everyone stops for tea time. But tea time is more than just tea; it is a small meal that prevents you from getting peckish before your actual dinner. As someone who loves to eat a little bit every few hours, this tradition was eagerly adopted by yours truly.

To learn, we signed up for High Tea at some fabulously posh hotel in Hyde Park. While I cannot remember the name of the hotel, I will never forget my first Tea Time. There were scones with clotted cream, biscuits (which aren't biscuits at all, but butter cookies), a few small cucumber sandwiches, and tea. Delicious, hot, aromatic, insanely good tea.

The tea sommelier coached us in the finer points of making and enjoying tea. I learned that one should never cradle the mug in their hands. I learned that one should never blow on tea to cool it. I learned you poured milk into the bottom of the cup and then poured tea over that. You could use milk or lemon, but never both at the same time. Black tea, the kind served most often at Tea Time, is steeped at 200° Fahrenheit for three minutes exactly. Each kind of tea varies slightly in the perfect temperature for the water and how long it should steep.

In my yoga studio 20 years later, I have a hot water button on my water bubble, making it possible to drink hot tea all day long. Irrespective of having hot water at my disposal, however, the sweet steeping spot for all teas is three to five minutes and for me, it's the steeping time that makes tea magical. The beauty of making a "cuppa" is that it takes time for the flavor to permeate the hot water.

And those precious few moments have become a mindfulness practice for me. As my tea steeps, I take a break from my day and try to just enjoy the steeping of my tea. I regularly break all the rules I learned at High Tea, cradling my mug to enjoy the warmth of the cup in my hands and blowing gently on it to release the aroma of the tea. I try to fully immerse myself in the experience of my cuppa. I've done this for so long that, like Pavlov's dogs, I've trained my body to take a long, deep breath every time I smell tea, even if I'm drinking it while teaching a class or waiting in the pick-up line. In this way, tea has become both a Digest and an Invite in my life, helping me to be both healthier and more present.

A Toddy for Your Body

- I mug decaffeinated tea
- Juice from ½ lemon
- 2 tsp honey (preferably local)
- 1 shot top shelf Kentucky bourbon

This recipe came from Erin's grandma, who swore that a "toddy for your body" would cure most ails. While we try to keep it for those times we feel a cold coming on, we can say it's been a balm for many hard knocks in our lives!

Alcohol

And having mentioned toddies, it's only right that we move onto the health benefits of drinking alcohol. But remember, we're talking moderation again. Enjoying the occasional drink responsibly has been shown to make your ticker stronger, gray matter sharper, and your dance moves more epically awesome. But we all know the risks of over-imbibing. And you certainly don't have to drink to be healthy. But we feel there is room for alcohol in a well-balanced wellness plan.

Research states that women may enjoy one drink per day to reap the health benefits. Andra follows this advice to the letter, enjoying exactly one craft beer each night. Erin prefers to drink only a few nights a week, but prefers two glasses of red wine (or one really great shot of bourbon).

2

Refined Sugar

Sugars are found naturally in fruits, vegetables, milk, and milk products. These foods contain the proper enzymes your body needs to digest them. Foods such as cakes, cookies, crackers, and cereal have all had sugars added. All of these sugars can be converted in your body to glucose (or blood sugar) which your cells "burn" for energy.

Added sugar is the leading food additive in the U.S. Most Americans eat almost 500 nutritionally empty calories of sugar daily! Numerous studies show that sugar, more than any other ingredient in the diet, is driving the increase in lifestyle diseases. When the low-fat guidelines first came out in the 90's, food manufacturers removed the fat from foods but added a whole bunch of sugar instead to make them palatable. But as bad as that was, they also managed to condition our taste buds in the process.

Remember our wellness bank account? The energy you get from sugar is mortgaged energy because more nutrients are needed to process it. Sugar literally eats up the nutrients you need to stay vibrant and healthy. It is an anti-nutrient ogre!

Myth: "Natural" sugars are better than refined sugar.

Truth: Honey, agave nectar, and coconut sugar are still forms of sug-

ar. While they are marketed as healthier alternatives to refined sugar, they still contain roughly the same amount of calories and are metabolized the same way as white sugar. Sugar is something we need to eat in moderation. Period.

We're not talking about fruit here though! Fruit does contain natural sugars, but also vitamins, minerals, and tons of awesome antioxidants. Plus, it's often packaged in a skin of fiber, which slows the absorption of fructose (the sugar found in fruit) into our bloodstream. Fruit is a real food and a real boon in your diet. So nosh on. If you like to drink your fruit, be sure to blend rather than juice as you don't want to separate the sugar from the fiber!

With over 29 million Americans currently suffering from diabetes, sugar is a beast we have got to wrangle down. If sugar is your personal struggle, try eating more high-quality protein. Sugar cravings are often a result of a protein deficiency.

Ghrelin is a hormone produced mainly in the stomach. Sugar elevates ghrelin levels, so your brain starts craving more sugar. If you're hungry (often from a lack of protein), cells containing ghrelin move from the stomach to the brain and tell you that not only are you famished, you need a big pile of CRAP right this very second! Protein keeps ghrelin levels balanced. Aim for less than 25 grams (6 teaspoons) of sugar and half of your body weight in protein (in grams) each day.

Stress makes us crave sugar as well. Cortisol is another hormone that spikes when we're anxious or stressed out. Elevated cortisol levels make us crave sugary, fatty, processed CRAP. Elevated cortisol and ghrelin together encourage belly fat, the kind of fat that strangles our internal organs and sets us up for the dreaded "lifestyle diseases" like heart disease, diabetes, and stroke. We'll talk more about cravings later in the chapter.

Refined sugar is a negative double whammy because it makes us feel and look old through a process call glycation. Glycation, over time, causes protein fibers to become stiff and misshapen. The proteins in skin most prone to glycation are the same ones that make us look beautiful, namely collagen and elastin. When those proteins connect with sugar molecules, they show up as wrinkles and loose, saggy skin.

Researchers in food labs are paid vast amounts of money to create foods with super tastes. They take something that's already sweet (like a donut), and they add unnecessary sugars, salt, and extra fat to light up taste buds all over your tongue. These fatty, sugary foods release chemicals called opioids into our bloodstream. Opioids bind to receptors in our brains and give us fleeting feelings of mild bliss. This euphoria makes us think our brain is thanking us for the donut and drives us to eat another. Then when we eat real food that is actually sweet (like a tangerine), we don't register its sweetness because it's too subtle. Our brains have been trained to want the food created in a lab. It's better to eat as little sugar as possible to retrain your brain into desiring real food.

If you must sweeten your coffee or tea, try some local honey. Locally produced honey is the least refined sugar out there. It contains pollen spores picked up by the bees from local plants and this introduces a small amount of the allergen into your system to activate your immune system. Over time, you can build up your natural immunity against these allergens. Plus, it activates serotonin and has been used for centuries to treat depression. The ancient Romans used honey to sweeten breads believed to increase happiness. Ceramic jars containing honey that is about 5,500 years old were recently discovered in a tomb in the Eurasian country of Georgia! But honey is still fructose (sugar), so be mindful and moderate!

> **Journal Prompt**: What refined sugars do you regularly consume? Become a label detective and find out where sugar is lurking in your fridge or pantry! Make

a list of the worst culprits and see how many you can replace with healthier, natural alternatives.

Some of the most common offenders include: agave syrup, beet sugar, cane sugar, caramel, corn syrup, date sugar, dextrose, ethyl maltol, fructose, galactose, glucose, high fructose corn syrup (HFCS), honey, juice concentrate, lactose, maltose, maltodextrin, maltose, molasses, sorghum and sucrose.

Replace the Sugar in Your Diet with Protein

When you're craving sugar, choose high quality protein instead. Proteins are an important part of your bones, muscles, and skin. In fact, proteins are in every living cell in your body. The word protein comes from the Greek protos, meaning "first" or "essential" and they are certainly that. Inside cells, proteins perform many functions. They help to break down food for energy, build new structures, and break down toxins.

In his great book *The China Study*, Dr. Colin Campbell explains how proteins are built. In order for protein to be constructed by the human body, a chain of 20 amino acids must be formed. It is helpful to think of the protein chain as a string of brightly colored beads and each amino acid is assigned its own unique color. Eleven of these amino acids are formed naturally in the human body (called non-essential) and nine must be consumed through our food (called essential).

Think of animal flesh as a necklace with all 9 essential color beads (amino acids). Plant meals tend to only have 6 or 7 colors, so it's harder to make the complete necklace. But your strand of amino acid beads doesn't have to be built with just one food at a time and you don't even need to build a complete strand all at one meal! If at one meal you are missing a few beads of lysine, you can make up for it in your next meal or two and have no issues. Since most plant-based foods are only missing one or two of the essential amino acids, it's not hard to create complete proteins.

So How Much Protein Do I Need?

The US Department of Agriculture currently recommends that all men and women over the age of 19 should get at least .37 grams of protein per pound of body weight per day.

Since we will later encourage you to strength train, we suggest you get about .5 grams of protein per pound of body weight per day.

This is what is suggested for athletes and make no mistake, you are an athlete! If you weigh 140 pounds, then you need 70 grams of high quality protein each day. But don't worry about counting grams of protein. Just eat a little protein at each meal in the form of eggs, wild-caught seafood, grass-fed lean and clean meats, vegetables, legumes, nuts, seeds, and powdered protein. You'll also be thrilled to learn that protein has a high thermogenic effect (meaning it boosts your metabolism). You burn about 30% of the calories the food contains during digestion!

What about Dairy?

Dairy is extremely acid forming (see the pH discussion below) and creates a lot of inflammatory mucous in the body. The body then spends its energy getting rid of the mucous any way it can. Sickeningly high amounts of hormones, antibiotics, and other toxins are found in most dairy products and your liver must work overtime to process them.

So how do you get enough calcium? This is a long-misunderstood piece of the nutrition puzzle. Dairy products do contain calcium, but animal proteins, sugars, hormones, and a substantial amount of fat and cholesterol accompany them.

Calcium is instrumental in regulating the body's pH balance (by keeping down inflammation levels in the body). When we eat dairy products, it creates inflammation. Consequently, calcium is leached from bones and teeth to buffer the acidic pH. But, once in the bloodstream, calcium isn't reabsorbed back into the bones. It's far better to get your calcium from "greens and beans" like kale, collards, arugula, broccoli, garbanzos, or soybeans.

There are a few exceptions. One is whey protein. The overall top food for maximizing your glutathione is high-quality whey protein. We talk more about this in the recipe section.

Another exception is goat or feta cheese. Yay, cheese! The great news is you can easily digest both goat and sheep milk cheeses because the fat molecules are smaller and their casein (protein) is similar to human breast milk. Milk from cows contains casein proteins our bodies find extremely hard to break down. The last form of dairy we promote is yogurt or kefir (goat or sheep milk yogurt inoculated with kefir grains to ferment).

Greek yogurt is strained more times than traditional yogurt to remove more whey. As a result, Greek yogurt is thicker and has more protein than regular yogurt and a higher amount of probiotics (good bacteria). Most regular yogurts have been homogenized so aggressively that the heat kills off most of the probiotics.

A healthy digestive tract contains a balance of both good and bad bacteria. A diet full of CRAP kills off many of the helpful bacteria, allowing the harmful bacteria to run amok. Redwood Hill Farms makes a high quality goat yogurt that is high in live cultures and available in many grocery stores. If your store doesn't carry it, don't be ashamed to ask them to do so! Our local supermarket has stocked goat dairy, alfalfa sprouts, and grass-fed butter simply because we asked them to!

Carnivore or Vegetarian?

Are you surprised to hear two yoginis suggesting that you eat meat? We're advocates of having some animal flesh in your diet, but only as long as you are really conscious of its source. Modern farming practices are what give most meat its deserved bad rap. Milk, cheese, farmed meat, and eggs from grain-fed chickens are a completely different food today than something our ancestors encountered a million years ago. Grain-fed animal products contain a sickeningly high amount of pesticide residue, growth hormones, and antibiotics. And aside from all of the nasty contained in this meat, the average American eats over 250 pounds of the stuff each year! This is entirely too much.

Erin's Edition:

I was raised a vegetarian. My Presbyterian/Buddhist/Hippie parents were ethically opposed to eating "anything with a face", though that rule was flexible when it came to creatures of the sea. Perhaps we cannot discern a scallop's face, but it is still a living being, right? Anyway, my folks are still strict non-meat eaters. I even became a vegan for a very (very) short time. And not only did I never miss meat, it made me a bit queasy to see it prepared and consumed.

So nobody was more surprised than me when I was pregnant and starting craving bacon! I'm not even sure I knew what bacon tasted like, but I wanted a BELT (very specifically, a BLT wouldn't do, it needed to be topped with a fried egg). But having lived my whole life shunning meat, it was important to me that I bridged the distance between my thoughts and actions. If I was going to eat meat, I would only do so mindfully, choosing sustainable meat that supported small farmers. Meat from small farms has more nutritional benefits and supporting small farms is aligned with my ethics.

I am surrounded these days by high-quality meat. Andra raises chickens, so there are always fresh eggs (and sometimes fried chicken when the hens get too old or lazy to produce). Those chickens are fed our table scraps, so it's a wonderful way to recycle.

Our next-door neighbor has a 300-acre bison farm. The bison at Blackfish Farm that I talk to over the fence on my morning woggles are the same ones in the tacos my family cooks on the weekends. Michael Pollan charges us to be "ecological detectives". Well, the mystery here is easily solved.

This compassionate food chain starts in the sun and moves in a direct line to the grass to the bison and then to me. No antibiotics, hormones, or cruelty necessary. This isn't CAFO agribusiness stripping our environment of its most precious resources. CAFOs (commercial animal feedlot operations) raise and maintain animals in confined situations on a small area of land. Feed is brought to the animals rather than allowing the animals to graze.

Blackfish is a small farm run by people who respect the earth and feel blessed to do what they do. These bison are happy animals, frolicking over the hills and playing in the pond. This is a farm of the kind that built this country, before farmers were forced to plant genetically modified high-yield plants or expand their livestock population just to make ends meet.

I've personally found that it is possible to have an occasional meat-based meal in my diet without trashing my ideals. Meat here and there makes me feel grounded and strong. If you choose to eat meat, choose the highest quality meat you can buy and do so mindfully.

Andra's Addition:

My meat and dietary journey is very different from Erin's. I was not raised a vegetarian but more of an omnivore. Well, as omnivore as one can be in a small southern town during the 70s and 80s. My mother cooked all of our meals and they were nearly always delicious, the exceptions coming during her occasional experimentations!

But the vast majority of what we ate was wholesome, southern and homemade. We always ate together laughing and enjoying each other's company. Being an only child, there were only three of us to feed so I didn't help with actual cooking and there was always plenty. My efforts were mostly relegated to setting the table, chopping things, and cleaning up after.

We didn't really think about the ethical treatment of the food we ate or the environmental acquisition costs, we just ate good homemade food. The only rules were that you had to eat what Zella (isn't that an awesome name?) cooked and she hated to waste anything. As a result, I'll try anything at least once and one of my current official titles at my house is the "Queen of Leftovers," just ask my kids!

There was very little processed food and always a variety of meat, fruit and vegetables that were featured on our table each week. We ate healthy, real food. Because snacking was light, we were hungry and ready to eat each meal. We were all busy with whatever, came together to eat and then went on about our way until the next meal. I know I sound like an old grouch, but it was a simpler food time then.

As I've grown older, food has gotten significantly more complicated. What most people put on their plates is very different from what graced the tables in my childhood. The majority of the food and drinks we consume are full of junk, huge environmental costs and clearly not making us healthier. Plus, we all seem very confused about exactly what we should be eating. I hear it, see it and live it every day. It's frustrating and simultaneously disheartening.

Other than using "vegetarianism" to mask a college eating disorder, I have always eaten meat regularly. I say "vegetarianism" in quotation marks because it was a sham, really. My real vegetarian friends would roll their eyes at "vegetarian" me back then. But as I got older and started a family of my own, I slowly began to think about what was going into our mouths and nourishing our bodies. Sometimes I thought about it more and took action, sometimes I was exhausted and busy and said "to hell with it" and we ate crap! Slowly, the good action started to exceed the crap and I made an astounding observation. I felt better when I ate real food! Let me say that another way to reinforce my point…I feel better when I eat real food!

At home, I am as busy as any other wife, mother and self-employed person on this beautiful earth. I strive every day and every meal to consume and feed my family the healthiest items possible. My meals and cooking are simple and basic; in fact they seem to actually get simpler each year. Good, tasty real food is actually easy if you take some time and learn how to cook it. I have learned that less in food preparation and cooking is truly better and healthier. Most weeks I do a great job at our food, but some weeks I don't. When we have those weeks, I think about all the good healthy meals that have gone before and try a little harder to do a better job next week. That's all any of us can really do. Have some grace and keep trying!

Here are a couple of delicious ways we fulfill our protein requirements both with and without meat.

Quinoa Buddha Bowl

Quinoa is a plant-based complete protein, meaning it contains all 9 essential amino acids. We bet you remember now that of the 20 different amino acids that can form a protein, there are nine that the body can't produce on its own. These are the essential amino acids - we need to eat them because we can't make them ourselves. Quinoa is a perfect way to get protein without eating animal flesh. We bet you'd be surprised to learn that botanically, quinoa is related to beets, chard and spinach! In fact, the leaves can be eaten as well as the grains. It's closer to a vegetable than a grain and is gluten-free.

We eat this over and over and never tire of it. A Buddha Bowl is a great way to use any veggies you have on hand. We've used spinach, butternut squash, tomatoes, avocados, whatever! A handful of dried cranberries or almonds can dress it up too. We like to make a big mess of quinoa in the rice cooker to use all week (one cup quinoa to two cups water). And here's a quick tip - massaging the kale breaks down the cellulose and makes it easier on your digestive tract!

- 1 cup quinoa
- 1 bunch kale, washed, chopped, and massaged
- 1 tsp olive or coconut oil
- 1/4 cup crumbled goat cheese or feta cheese
- sea salt and pepper

Cook or reheat quinoa in a pan over low heat. Add the kale and oil to warm. Transfer to a bowl and add the cheese, salt, and pepper.

It is entirely possible to fulfill your protein requirements choosing nuts and seeds over animal flesh. Erin did it for years, though she chooses to eat some meat these days.

Erin's Bison Tacos

We live next to a grass-fed bison farm, so we always have incredible meat. This guacamole with some low-fat ground bison wrapped in a whole-wheat tortilla makes the perfect taco. Dice some lettuce and tomatoes to let people build their own. Sriracha is a must for us. You will NOT miss the cheese or sour cream in traditional tacos.

- 1 lb of ground bison
- 2 tbsp olive oil
- ¼ tsp garlic powder
- ¼ tsp crushed red pepper flakes
- 1½ tsp ground cumin
- 1 tsp sea salt
- 1 tsp black pepper
- whole-wheat tortillas
- ½ cup of red or green cabbage
- ¼ cup cilantro chopped
- ¼ cup prepared salsa (or diced tomatoes)

- sriracha
- guacamole (recipe below)

Heat pan on medium with olive oil. Add bison, cook until done. About 7-10 minutes. Meat should be slightly pink. Because bison is low in fat, it will get tough if you overcook it. Add spices. Place tortilla on plate and spoon meat on top of tortilla. Add desired toppings on top of meat.

Guacamole

- 2 avocados, mashed
- salsa (or fresh tomatoes) to taste
- juice from 1 lime
- handful cilantro, finely chopped
- sea salt

Mix it all together. Enjoy.

3

Artificial Colors

Did you know that about 15 million pounds of petroleum-based dyes are used in food each year? Gross, right? Most dyes are added to processed food to make them appear like a healthy food. But ingesting these dyes has been linked to tumors and cancers. Instead of eating fake colors, eat from the Rainbow.

Eat the Rainbow Instead!

Choosing a variety of fruits and vegetables will ensure you get the proper vitamins and minerals in your diet. Plants derive their colors from various phytochemicals found in them. For example, yellow and orange fruits and vegetables are abundant in vitamins C and A. Green fruits and veggies are high in vitamins K, B, and E. Blue and purple produce is high in vitamins C and K.

Vitamins

Vitamins are substances found in foods that your body needs for growth and health. There are 13 vitamins your body needs. They are Vitamin A, B (includes thiamine, riboflavin, niacin, pantothenic acid, biotin, B-6, B-12 and, folate), C, D, E, and K. Each vitamin has a specific job.

If you are eating a nutrient-rich, colorful array of fruits and vegetables, then you are fulfilling your daily requirements for vitamins.

Minerals

Like vitamins, minerals are substances found in food that your body needs for growth and health. There are two kinds of minerals: macrominerals and trace minerals. Macrominerals are minerals your body needs in larger amounts. They include calcium, phosphorus, magnesium, sodium, potassium, and chloride. Your body needs just small amounts of trace minerals. These include iron, copper, iodine, zinc, fluoride, and selenium. Minerals occur naturally in non-living things like rocks and metal ores. Plants get their essential minerals from the soil in which they grow. We get essential minerals by including plants in our diet.

Myth: I take a multivitamin, so I've covered all my bases when it comes to vitamins and minerals.

Truth: Our bodies were designed to extract nutrients from real food. We most easily absorb those nutrients from the "food matrix", a term used to describe the bioavailability of nutrients based on the molecular structure of natural foods (as opposed to lab-made food products). For instance, the synthetic B-6 used in multivitamins is not molecularly the same as B-6 found in real foods like nuts, seeds, and fish. Our bodies are consequently not sure what to do with the lab-created vitamin. Is it a friend or a foe? If our digestive tract doesn't view it as "food," it's likely going to be sent out as waste. This means those expensive supplements are simply creating expensive urine.

There is medical evidence suggesting that multivitamins offer little or no health benefits, and some studies suggest that high doses of vitamins might even cause harm. This "nutritional insurance plan" can be too much of a good thing, as we still don't know what consuming more than 100% of the RDA of certain vitamins and minerals does to the body. The exception is when you're pregnant or deficient in a specific thing (based on blood work). Erin takes vitamin D each winter because September blood work almost always shows a deficiency (it's real cloudy around these parts about 6 months of the year).

Many vegetables are now mineral-deficient because over-farming has depleted the soil. This is why it's an investment in your health to buy organic produce.

The Environmental Working Group is an organization dedicated to protecting human health and the environment. Their annual Dirty Dozen List refers to the 12 foods that contain the most pesticides relative to other produce items. If these foods contain pesticide residue, you can bet the soil is also deficient in naturally occurring minerals. The 2014 list includes apples, strawberries, grapes, celery, peaches, spinach, sweet bell peppers, nectarines, cucumbers, cherry tomatoes, snap peas and potatoes. With these items specifically, buy organic whenever possible.

Beans and Greens Rainbow Soup

- 3 14-ounce cans vegetable broth
- 1 15-ounce can tomato puree
- 1 15-ounce can Great Northern beans, drained and rinsed
- ½ cup uncooked quinoa
- ½ cup finely chopped onion
- 1 cup sliced carrots
- 3 cup cauliflower florets
- 1 14-ounce can light coconut milk
- handful fresh basil, chopped
- Sea salt and pepper to taste
- 2 garlic cloves, chopped
- 8 cups coarsely chopped fresh spinach or kale leaves

In a stockpot, combine everything except the greens. Cover, almost bring to a boil and then cook on low for 20-30 minutes. Just before serving, stir in spinach or kale.

Eating the Rainbow Also Ensures You Get Enough Fiber

Fibers are carbohydrates that your body cannot digest. They pass through your body without being broken down into sugars. Even though your body does not get energy from fiber, you still need fiber to stay healthy. Fiber also binds to cholesterol-rich bile acids in the digestive tract and removes these acids from the body to keep your cholesterol levels in check. Fiber helps push food through the intestines, which helps prevent constipation and it also absorbs water to keep the waste in your colon soft and moving easily.

Foods high in fiber include fruits, vegetables, beans, peas, nuts, seeds, and whole grains. Refined grains (CRAP like white rice or boxed pasta) lack all the original nutrients but still contain all the original calories. Women should aim for 20-25 grams of fiber each day. But again, you needn't do math to eat well. Just include fiber-rich foods in your daily diet. If you're pooping every day, you're probably getting enough fiber. Fiber creates a sense of fullness so it helps us eat more of the right foods and less CRAP. The best fiber is insoluble fiber from fruits and veggies.

Think of vegetables as Diana Ross. Protein and carbs are those poor Supremes. The veggies are the diva and should get your main focus. The protein and carbohydrates have a smaller, supporting role.

Your plate should be as colorful as possible. Eating a rainbow diet means you get the highest assortment of phytonutrients, antioxidants, and fiber.

> **Journal Prompt**: What can choosing real foods do for me? What dietary choices make me feel my very best? Why do I resist these choices? What small changes can I make to cultivate these choices on a daily basis?

One huge mistake people make is putting together a beautiful, colorful salad and then drowning it in store-bought dressings filled with high-fructose corn syrup and unhealthy fats like vegetable, soybean, sunflower and corn oils. Skip the store bought salad dressings and make your own. They're really easy and super delicious!

The directions for all of these dressings are exactly the same! Just dump the ingredients together in a jelly jar and screw the lid on tightly. Shake vigorously and you're set. Plus, you can leave them on the countertop all week without having to refrigerate!

Honey Mustard Dressing

- 2 tsp (good quality) olive oil
- 4 tsp white wine vinegar
- 4 tsp (local) honey
- 4 tsp Dijon mustard

Strawberry Vinaigrette

- 1/4 cup fresh strawberries (blended)
- 1/2 tsp (high quality) olive oil
- 1/2 tsp balsamic vinegar
- sea salt and pepper
- pinch of dried tarragon
- 1/4 tsp honey

Hoisin-Sesame Dressing

- 1/3 cup coconut oil
- 3 tsp rice vinegar
- 2 tsp hoisin sauce
- 1 tsp toasted sesame oil
- 1 tsp toasted sesame seeds
- 1 scallion, minced

The Truth about Gluten

Gluten-free diets have become all the rage of late and have been trending constantly over the last couple of years. Gluten, which gives elasticity to dough, helping it rise and keep its shape, is created when two molecules, glutenin and gliadin, interact and form a bond. It often gives the final product a chewy consistency. Gluten adds mouth feel to foods, so your body feels like it has been fed. Gluten-free varieties of the same foods often have added sugar and fat to make them tasty.

Gluten itself doesn't offer nutritional benefits. But the whole grains that contain gluten do. Whole grains contain the whole seed: the nutrient-rich germ, the fiber-rich bran, and the endosperm. Ingesting the whole seed allows us to get all of the fiber. They're rich in an array of vitamins and minerals like vitamin B, iron, and fiber. Studies show that whole grain foods may help lower risk of heart disease, type-2 diabetes, and some forms of cancer.

For those without celiac disease, a gluten-free diet can actually lack vitamins, minerals, and fiber. Plus, the starches in wheat support healthy digestive bacteria. In fact, recent studies from the National Institute of Health suggest those on a gluten-free diet have lower levels of healthy gut bacteria. Damage your healthy gut bacteria and your small intestine will struggle to properly digest everything you eat.

So what's with all the so-called experts bashing gluten? Generally, the people encouraging you to completely rid your body of grains took research based on very excessive amounts of refined grains and applied it to the eating of any or all grains. No one is going to eat the amount of grains the poor rats in these studies were force-fed!

Gluten can create an inflammatory response, so too much isn't good. Much of the wheat we eat today has been milled into white flour, which has tons of gluten but few vitamins or nutrients. We can temper this by eating bread we've made at home (or by buying homemade bread), for less gluten.

Up until 25 years or so ago, bread was made using a sourdough process based on lacto-fermentation. The process was slow, so when modern yeast became available, sourdough breads became less common. Now research shows us that lacto- fermentation of wheat has the potential to drastically reduce gluten levels. The take away? Baking bread yourself is far superior to buying loaves off the grocery shelf. Don't bake? Support your local artisanal bakery or CSA (Community Supported Agriculture). Good homemade bread with real butter and honey is delicious but like anything, be sure to enjoy it in moderation.

> *Myth: Carbohydrates are the devil's work!*
>
> *Truth: We are so sick and tired of defending the embattled carbohydrate. We are not talking about defending Wonder Bread but complex carbohydrates like whole wheat bread, brown rice and real homemade pasta (yes, that's OK). Carbohydrates are an important part of eating properly, but get a bad rap because if we eat too much of the wrong kind and are sedentary, then our body stores them as fat. Carbohydrates are the body's favorite energy source and in choosing complex or "good" carbs, coupled with protein, fruits/veggies and*

moving your body, you simply can't go wrong!

4

Processed Products

This one's really easy. Replace processed food with real food. Choose real food that is easily and quickly digested. Remember our favorite Michael Pollan quote? Chemists are paid large sums of money to create long-lasting, artificially delicious food.

Check labels. If you can't pronounce it, chances are your body doesn't truly know how to digest it. In fact, the best foods won't even have a label!

Chemicals aren't nutrients. They don't satisfy hunger, they're addictive, and they make you gain weight. Digestion takes up between 50-75% of our total energy at any one time. The less energy you spend digesting, the more energy you have to build muscle, build collagen, grown strong hair and nails, and stay radiant. Let the mirror be your guide! Under-eye circles, acne, brittle hair, and too many wrinkles reveal a body overtaxed from digestion with overall stagnant flow.

Keep It Simple, Stupid!

We've made eating far too complicated. If you're eating real food, your body will respond by settling into its happy place. There is no need to count calories, use the glycemic index, or use a point system. And there's absolutely no requirement for a scale. In fact, we want you to break up with that dumb piece of plastic for good! It's a toxic relationship that drains your self-esteem and gives you nothing positive in return.

A number on a scale cannot define how beautiful, talented, smart, successful, compassionate, and funny you are!

Your weight is not a good tool to measure your success. Your weight fluctuates too much throughout the month based on hormonal fluctuations, salt consumption, and water retention. You might weigh yourself once a month, just to notice trends. But weighing yourself all the time can make you go crazy. That stupid number could go up or down five pounds over the course of a single day!

We want you to measure success based on how you feel as time passes. A number on a scale tells you nothing about how healthy you are.

Shift your focus from how you look to how you feel. Follow the Four and we promise you'll feel great!

1. Replace soda with water, coffee, tea, and moderate amounts of alcohol.
2. Replace refined sugar with protein.
3. Replace artificial colors with real colors by eating the rainbow.
4. Replace processed foods with real foods that have pronounceable ingredients.

Now that you've mastered the four basic eating guidelines, here are a few other things to chew on.

What We Can Learn From the Japanese

The Okinawan people are known for living long, healthy lives. The Standard Japanese Diet (SJD) is much like that of the Mediterranean Diet, with its emphasis on daily movement, vegetables, whole grains, fruits, legumes and fish with limited amounts of lean meats and processed foods. One difference is the Okinawan emphasis on **hara hachi bu**. This is the Japanese practice of eating until you are 80% full.

It takes your brain about 20 minutes to fully register your fullness. Unfortunately, most of us are overstuffed by then!

You can start by ordering lunch portions at dinner or using smaller plates. You might feel hungry at first, but it takes 15-20 meals for your stomach to get used to less food. Be patient!

Why Diets Fail

Diet is, to us, a four-letter word. At any given time, over 100 million Americans are on a diet or eating plan. That's almost a third of the American population. If diets worked, we wouldn't be some of the fattest people on earth! Diets ultimately fail because they approach food from a place of right and wrong.

Living from a place of deprivation and guilt robs us of our beautiful, radiant light.

Calorie counting and deprivation is not for us. We are both hungry girls who need a lot of calories to exist. A mindfulness practice has helped us fuel our bodies properly with lots of clean food. Dump the deprivation!

Ever had a girlfriend blow off a dinner date because she was dieting and built herself a jail where bread or wine was forbidden? Ever worried about an event because you were unsure what you should (could) eat? Stop being so rigid!

Remember that wellness account? Some foods are a deposit (they give you energy) and some are a withdrawal (they sap your energy). But that doesn't mean that you can eat the latter. For example, we both share a passion for a good kettle chip. We can mindfully choose to eat them occasionally, as long as we are mindful that it isn't crediting our energy account. But when we do indulge, we enjoy the hell out of them.

Common sense tells us that there is no NEVER. Diets just focus on NEVERS and SHOULD NOTS and that is not the headspace we want in live in!

Add to that the fact that popular diets such as Weight Watchers, The Zone, and Atkins have an over 80% failure rate. This means that for every person who loses weight on these programs, there are four people who don't. And over three quarters of those people that did lose weight will put some of it back on. Why does this happen? For one thing, most of these programs focus on restricting calories or by completely outlawing certain foods like bread or alcohol. Thus, they are not maintainable in the long-term. People are overwhelmed with too many rules and throw in the towel after a few weeks of deprivation.

Our bodies are designed to be fed and too few calories make us grouchy and sick. Plus, a calorie is not a calorie (as you already know from our wellness account discussion). 100 calories of CRAP is not the same as 100 calories of nutrient-rich food. The CRAP taxes your digestive system and gives no real nourishment. Food satisfies our craving by providing actual vitamins and minerals that we need to function well.

Diets also rarely take into consideration that human beings are vastly different when it comes to our genes, environments and thoughts. So no ONE diet could possibly work for everyone!

Aren't you tired of the so-called diet experts who proclaim they alone have figured out the secret to lasting weight loss and vital health? And did you ever notice how often those claims come packaged with a plan or item they want you to buy?

Do you choose to be a part of the for-profit diet industry or do you want to be in charge of a for-you life? We want to empower you to take charge of your own health by showing you that you can do it without being a part of that industry and without spending hundreds of dollars on diet plan memberships and pre-packaged food. Everyone requires a different eating plan to stay healthy and balanced. There is no simple, easy fix. You must figure out the perfect, unique equation that works for you.

We all know that gal who swears by the diet she's on. She's lost weight and she can't stop talking about it. But often this gal is "skinny fat," a term that describes someone who has a normal body weight, but is deficient in nutrients.

"Skinny fat" people believe that being thin is the ultimate goal. We know it's not. Being healthy is the ultimate goal!

Humans are born with between 5-10 billion fat cells. Healthy adults have about 25-30 billion fat cells. Fat cells expand when people consume more calories than they can burn. During weight loss, the cells shrink. But the fat cells never go away (without liposuction, which we do not recommend). The number of cells stays fairly consistent - we are just constantly either shrinking or expanding them.

But people who yo-yo diet have a tendency to add fat cells when they gain back weight. This is bad news because now they have more fat cells screaming to be fed. People who are obese can have up to 100 billion fat cells! Find a happy weight that is appropriate for your unique genetic make-up and then let go of all the calorie counting. Eat clean and your cells will do the rest to keep you where you need to be.

Journal Prompt: Food journal. Keep a food journal for three days. Write down every single thing that passes your lips. Note all beverages too. This is simply data collection - most people are sincerely surprised by what they're consuming. It is not about feeling shameful or guilty. It is not to count your calories. It's just to see where the crap is creeping in and how you might make tiny changes to feel better overall.

A huge surprise for Erin was her coffee, which she took her entire adult life "sweet and blonde, just like me." One tablespoon of sugar and two ounces of milk each day over a year adds up to more than 22 cups of sugar and 91 cups of milk each year. That's a lot of inflammation! Switching out her milk and sugar for a spoonful of coconut oil was easy for her because the change in taste was palatable to her.

Now Andra wouldn't give up cream in her morning coffee for any amount of money, so this would be an unsustainable thing to ask of her. Her insidious nutritional demon was high-fructose corn syrup lurking in the hot sauces and barbeque sauces in her fridge. Making her own, healthier versions was a quick and easy fix! All you need are a few basic ingredients, a jelly jar, and 60 seconds. She didn't sacrifice the tastes her family loves and improved everyone's overall health.

> The moral of these stories? Without our occasional food journals, we wouldn't have been aware of how change was necessary!

So I Can Change My Fat Into Muscle?

Sadly, no. This is one of the most misunderstood components of exercise. Fat and muscle are comprised of completely different tissues. A fat cell cannot turn into a muscle cell.

So where does fat go when we lose weight? Believe it or not, you actually exhale it! Remember that the fat cell doesn't disappear - you're simply shrinking it. If you monitor the atoms of a fat cell, we find that metabolized fat ends up as carbon dioxide, water and energy. So about 80% of it is exhaled out of your body. The other 20% is excreted through urine, feces, and sweat. Just another reason to learn to breathe well!

Will Following the Four Guidelines Get Rid of my Cellulite?

Women constantly ask us how they can rid their thighs of cellulite. Cellulite is that lumpy, dimpled flesh on the buttocks and thighs. Almost 90% of women will have some amount of cellulite in their life.

Imagine an old building that is surrounded by scaffolding. Between the skin and the subcutaneous fat, there lies a layer of connective tissue that acts like scaffolding on a crumbling building to hold the fat in place. Age, extra weight, hormones, or a genetic predisposition may affect the integrity of this scaffolding, allowing the fat to bulge up between weaker scaffolding sections. The scaffolding in women runs vertically (imagine metal poles drilled into a building to hold it up during repairs). Picture those crossed X's on really strong sections of scaffolding. That's the shape of the connective scaffolding in men; their scaffolding has more integrity, so less fat can bulge through.

There is currently no permanent cure for cellulite. But you can lessen the appearance of cellulite by eating clean, staying hydrated, and weight training, since strengthening muscle and tightening the connective tissues of the body will help maintain the integrity of your connective tissue scaffold.

Improving the blood flow around the area will also ensure that nutrients reach the surface area for healthy skin turnover. Estrogen keeps blood vessels flowing smoothly. But as we age, women make less estrogen (and, seemingly, more cellulite). Further, this is an area with less circulation generally.

Have you ever peeled off your stinky clothes after a workout and noticed that, even though you're sweating and hot all over, your buttocks remain cold and clammy to the touch? This is because there is a lot more fat, which is an inactive tissue with fewer blood vessels than muscle. So we need to pay special attention to this area to help the existing blood vessels do their best job. Dry brushing and body rolling (two things we discuss in the REST section) are proven ways to improve circulation in these areas.

How Dieting Damages Your Metabolism

When we think of diets, we think of calorie restriction and being hungry. We've all tried them and know they simply don't work and aren't sustainable. This is true for two reasons. The first reason is that diets operate in the world of extremes. Any eating plan that seems unrealistic and full of extremes is simply not sustainable.

We cannot function on reduced calories, eating very restricted foods, or eliminating entire food groups. Follow the Four to

nourish your body.

Diets are just not possible to sustain and you must adopt a long-range view of fitness and nutrition and an attitude of moderation to be successful. The other reason is that when you attempt these unsustainable diet methods, it actually damages your metabolism. It changes your body composition for the worse by decreasing the amount of lean muscle mass in your body while increasing the amount of fat. Dieting is just not as effective as eating clean, nutrient-rich food and choosing movements that will build muscle.

The good news is that you can rebuild the composition of your body to create lean muscle mass no matter how many times you have damaged your metabolism. The human body is amazing that way! You just have to retrain yourself to eat real, healthy foods and create gorgeous muscles. It's really as simple as that.

We want you to change the way you look at food, movement, and your body. We want you to focus on attainable, realistic goals that emphasize your health, not some pie-in-the-sky beauty ideal. If you're pear-shaped and overweight, when you lose weight you will simply be a smaller pear-shape! You cannot spot reduce using diet or exercise. But what we are offering you is so much more important.

Following the Four will help you squeeze every bit of life out of your days because you will feel your best You. The rest of your life will be the best of your life.

What About Cheating?

Nothing makes us angrier than a beautiful woman talking about how she's "cheating" on her diet by having a glass of wine or a slice of cake.

The whole idea of cheating implies eating is something for which we should feel guilty. It isn't.

Learn to be mindful and respond to your body's signals and there is no need to think of foods as "good" or "bad". Different foods serve different needs. Most of the time, we want you to eat to nourish your cells, but sometimes you must eat to nourish your soul. Pizza, beer, and cake won't destroy you, as long as they are eaten on special occasions and with mindfulness. If you're scarfing down slice after slice every day at lunch, then you've got a problem. You should feel empowered in your own life and know that you are the best judge of what you need to feel fabulous.

Be mindful, be moderate, and enjoy the hell out of an occasional slice of pie!

Life is a journey of moments to be savored. Don't be scared to enjoy something sweet every now and then. Remember most of our sugar intake is lurking in processed food. If you're eating less processed foods, it's OK to have a homemade dessert in moderation. In fact, you should savor and enjoy it! Take control of the food you buy and live your life already!

Andra's Favorite Dessert: Fruit Crisp

- 1 stick grass fed organic butter
- 1 cup cane sugar
- 1 cup self rising flour
- 1 cup organic whole milk
- 1 16-oz bag frozen blackberries (any frozen fruit could be used)

Preheat oven to 350°. In small bowl whisk the sugar, flour and milk until it becomes a smooth batter. Melt the stick of butter in a 9x13" glass casserole dish. Pour the batter into the butter but do not mix them together - let them mix as they will. Sprinkle the frozen blackberries into the batter/butter mixture and place in the oven to back for 1 hour. Enjoy with a little natural ice cream (should have less than 5 ingredients).

Erin's Favorite Dessert: Grilled Peaches with Bourbon Glaze and Yogurt

Grilling intensifies the sweetness of peaches. One of my favorite indulgences is a glass of top-shelf bourbon-I'm a Kentucky girl through and through. Pour a glass of bourbon (I prefer Woodford Reserve or Bulleitt) to enjoy the sunset while the grill heats.

- (2-inch) piece vanilla bean, split lengthwise
- 1 cup yogurt
- 6 tsp dark brown sugar, divided
- 1/4 tsp sea salt, divided
- 4 tsp bourbon
- ½ tsp vanilla extract
- 4 firm, ripe peaches, halved and pitted

Scrape seeds from vanilla bean into a medium bowl. Combine seeds, bean, yogurt, 2 tablespoons sugar, and a dash of salt. Let stand for 1 hour and discard bean.

Preheat grill. Combine remaining sugar, dash of salt, bourbon, and vanilla extract in a large bowl, stirring with a whisk. Add peaches and toss very gently. Arrange peaches, cavity side up, on grill (you should be able to hold your hand about an inch above the cooking grate for 3 to 4 seconds). Cook the peaches until grill marks show and the peaches are tender (but not falling apart). Turn peach halves over and drizzle cavities with reserved sugar mixture. Serve with yogurt and juices and, quite possibly, another glass of bourbon!

Eating When Stressed

Ayurveda offers a great rule of nourishment that suggests we never eat when we are upset, stressed out, or overly anxious.

It isn't enough to focus on what you're eating. You also have to focus on what's eating you.

If you're angry or frazzled, you will not digest your food well, regardless of what you eat. Stress is a major player in indigestion, IBS, ulcers, colitis, and heartburn. When we are calm and relaxed, enzymes and hormones governing digestion and absorption work at their peak performance. We'll talk about ways to engage the anabolic, relaxation response in the Rest section.

Cravings

When you switch from processed to more whole foods, your mind will resist terribly. You may feel deprived and frustrated that you continue to want fattening, processed foods. The idea of eating real food sounds great, but the reality of no CRAP bites the big one.

You have to change your mindset. Instead of saying no to fettuccine alfredo, say yes to udon noodles with broccoli. Instead of saying no to a head of romaine lettuce drenched in bleu cheese, say yes to beet salads with a little goat cheese.

Do it enough and eventually you'll find yourself becoming very discerning about what you agree to. You are not saying no to anything. But remember that what you promote, you permit. There isn't anything off limits in your life (except smoking, that's a deal breaker anyway you look at it). We just want you to be more discerning about what you agree to.

Erin's Edition:

I love to say yes to an occasional plate of hand-cut fries (my personal Achilles heel is a potato in a fry or chip mode). But if I say yes too frequently, I'm also saying yes to weight gain, bloating, acne, and, eventually, heart disease or high cholesterol. I'll say yes to an occasional glass of top shelf bourbon. But every night? That's agreeing to unhealthy spikes of blood sugar and a possible addiction. These are not yeses I can get behind. These yeses dilute my true path and become ways to numb myself to life instead of waking up to it.

Mindful Eating

We have one last piece of advice about nutrition but it's a biggie. In fact, if it's the only thing you take away from this book, we'll be happy. In our diet-obsessed culture, eating is often mindless. We either eat too quickly with no regard to how we feel as we eat or we eat from a place of guilt and punishment by labeling foods as "good" or "bad". We are in such a hurry most days that we often eat from a place of stress or anxiety and then misinterpret our brain's signals. We think we are hungry when really we might be thirsty, anxious, or simply tired.

Mindful eating is your new superpower!

Journal Prompt: Savor the moment. Slow down. Take a deep breath before you even sit down. This breath will help us be really present. How does the food look? What aromas do you notice? What do you hear? Observe the texture and temperature of your food. Be present and honor that nourishing yourself is a sacred practice.

Remember all those animals we share space with? We love to watch them eat. Both wild and domesticated animals eat when they are hungry and stop when they've had enough. The only clock they eat by is their internal body clock. We have that inner clock as well - we have just forgotten how to use it!

Halfway through your meal, set your fork down and take a few deep breaths again. Check in with the physical sensations and signals your body is sending you. Am I still hungry? Am I full? Am I thirsty? In yoga, we tell our students that if we can learn to hear the body whisper, we'll never have to hear it shout. The whispers tell us how something truly tastes or when we've had enough. The shouting comes with bloating, gas, and indigestion.

The quieter we are, the more we hear. ~Zen proverb

Slow down and be mindful when you eat. You are your own nutritional therapist. You alone know how energetic or depleted you feel when you eat certain foods. Eating is a natural, healthy, and pleasurable activity that nourishes both our cells and our souls. It allows people to connect to each other on a deep, lasting level.

Mindful eating is eating with intention and attention. Choose foods for both enjoyment and nourishment and then let it fuel the shiny life you crave!

Grocery List

We would encourage you to be a food snob. Start reading labels and choose the products that have the fewest number of unpronounceable ingredients. Turn your nose up at processed foods, chemically engineered food stuffs, soft drinks, and absolutely anything labeled low-fat or low-carb. That just means they shot that thing full of CRAP chemicals to make up for the taste they subtracted when taking out fat or carbohydrates.

When you find yourself in the grocery aisle full of processed CRAP, turn your nose right up in the air and walk on by. You're better than that. You deserve only the best and it'll be found in the periphery of the store. A sample grocery list follows on the next page. Take a photo on your smart phone so you always have it with you at the store.

Almond Milk
Coconut Milk
Protein powder
Chia seeds
Eggs
Plain Yogurt
Fresh Salmon (wild caught)
Clean and lean meat
Ground bison
Beans (dried or canned)
Tofu
Almond Butter
Peanut Butter
Cashews
Pistachios
Walnuts
Almonds
Quinoa
Oats (steel cut)
Sprouted Bread
Whole-wheat tortilla wraps

Goat cheese
Feta cheese
In-Season fruit
Frozen berries
Spinach
Mixed Baby Greens
Kale
Carrots
Peppers
Beets
Brussels sprouts
Broccoli (frozen)
Cauliflower (frozen)
Avocados*
Salsa
Cherry Tomatoes
Cucumbers
Zucchini
Lemons
Coconut Oil
Olive oil

White wine vinegar
Apple Cider Vinegar
Balsamic Vinegar
Dijon Mustard
Soy Sauce
Sriracha
Honey (local)
Cocoa powder
Dark chocolate
Cayenne Pepper
Turmeric
Himalayan Sea Salt
Ginger root (fresh)
Coffee
Herbal tea
Red wine

Erin's Edition:

Erin's Cooking Philosophy

Full disclosure here! I don't cook in the traditional sense. I just never fell in love with cooking. My husband is a great cook and really enjoys it, so he does the lion's share of food prep in our house. I'm sure you're asking yourself what kind of nutritional therapist doesn't like to cook? The answer is one who really likes to eat! But I do have a few go-to meals. My standards have fewer than 7 ingredients, are ready quickly, and often involve kale or avocadoes (two things I always have on hand).

Things you'll always find in my kitchen are avocados, goat yogurt, nuts, sprouted bread, kale, honey, apple cider vinegar, tea, and coconut oil. I can't live without my Vitamix, my small toaster oven, and my Global chef's knife.

Andra's Addition:

Andra's Cooking Philosophy

It is important to me that my family has hot, healthy, homemade meals and I am the primary cook in our home. Every weekend, I plan meals for the week. I shop for three homemade meals, one soup, a bean dish, and a meat dish. On Sundays, I make soup. On nights I teach yoga, my family heats up the soup I made. The other dishes I make are large enough that we can eat for two nights. In this way, no one comes home starving and eats CRAP out of the pantry. I've taught my children to make a few simple meals like scrambled eggs or vegetable panini.

Things you'll always find in my kitchen are eggs, canned beans, avocados, rice, frozen berries, yogurt, almond milk, coffee, and peanut butter. I can't live without my rice cooker, my panini maker, and my iron skillet.

Breakfast

Never skip breakfast! Skipping meals doesn't help you lose weight. Drops in blood sugar results in a release of cortisol, which breaks down tissues (like those muscles you worked so hard to build during your workouts) and slows your metabolism. Studies say that people who start the day with a protein-rich meal make healthier food choices the rest of the day!

Breakfast Shake

Glutathione, a tripeptide found inside every single cell in your body, is your body's most powerful antioxidant. It acts like flypaper for free radicals and toxins of all kinds. Proper glutathione levels are actually required so that the other antioxidants such as vitamins C, E, selenium and carotenoids, can be properly utilized within the body. Natural glutathione production is easily disrupted and stores can become quickly depleted by a poor diet, stress, medications, infections and other toxins.

Therefore, in a modern world that is often tumultuous and not that natural, taking special care to maintain proper glutathione levels in the body is really important.

- 1 scoop vanilla or chocolate whey protein powder (whatever brand you prefer, as long as it has less than 4 grams of sugar per serving)

- A handful of kale
  1 cup yields 132% K, 354% A, 89% C, 27% manganese, and %5 or more fiber, calcium, B6, iron, magnesium, omega-3 fats, B2 and protein!

- 1 tbsp Chia seeds
  One half ounce (about 1 tablespoon) contains 70 calories, 2 grams of protein, 4 grams fat, 6 grams carbohydrates and 6 grams of fiber, plus vitamins and minerals, including omega-4 fatty acids. That's a powerful tablespoon!

- ½-1 cup almond/coconut milk
  This yummy deliciousness contains MCFAs. MCFAs, or medium-chain fatty acids, are a type of saturated fat consisting of eight to 10 carbon atoms strung together in a row. Long-chain fatty acids, or LCFAs, contain 12 or more carbon atoms in a row and are more prevalent in meat and dairy products. MCFAs are more quickly metabolized than LCFAs.

- Handful Frozen Berries
  Frozen berries are just as nutritious (and in some cases higher in certain nutrients) than fresh berries. Berries of all types are rich in vitamin C and other antioxidants that help protect against cell damage that leads to diseases like cancer, heart disease, impaired vision, and age-related decline in both memory and motor skills. Freezing retains vitamin C content.

PART THREE
MOVE

Movement is amazing! We were designed by nature to move our bodies. We can run, walk, jump, scoot, dance, twirl, wave, hug, and make love.

Think back to yourself as a child. You didn't exercise. You played.

What were your favorite hobbies and activities back then? Consider all the different shapes your body took climbing trees, playing tag, catching fireflies, or roller skating. You were thrilled to see all the different ways your body could propel you through space. You didn't have to train certain parts of the body, as your daily activities kept you in game-day shape.

Then life happened. We're guessing you picked up a husband, career, or kids along the way. And your day became so filled with making lunches, school drop-offs, eight-hour work days, school pick-ups, dinner-making, laundry, housecleaning, and ten thousand other chores that movement was one thing that fell by the wayside. Now we're dealing with the law of inertia, which states that an object at rest will stay at rest until acted on by a moving force. You stopped moving regularly and it's really hard to get started again. But we promise that if you do, you'll be astounded at the amount of energy it will actually give you. We want you to fall in love again with movement.

The very best form of exercise is the one that you'll do.

It's that simple. Studies show that weight loss is linked more closely to whether a person sticks to their fitness routine than to what that routine is. A routine that you enjoy is more likely to lead to the long-term goals you are seeking. But you have to move! You've probably heard that 80% of weight loss comes from what we ingest and only 20% comes from exercise. This is true. We've read diet books that encourage you not to start an exercise program until after you've lost your desired amount of weight. This is crazy talk! That 20% is really powerful. Not only does lean muscle mass burn more calories at rest than fat, movement lowers your stress levels so that you can be more mindful in other areas of your life.

Movement increases the brain's production of a protein called brain-derived neurotropic factor (BDNF). This protein helps developing neurons to survive and promotes the growth of new ones. Think of BDNF as nourishment for your brain! In other words, when you work out, you're improving your mood, memory, and creativity.

Regular exercisers heal from injuries and illnesses eight times faster than couch potatoes. I bet you can guess why too. Oxygen inside kick-starts the lymphatic system and your skin sweats out tons of toxins.

Fitness traditionally includes the three pillars of strength, endurance, and flexibility. We would add a mind-body connection, because the first three without the fourth breeds injury and inefficient results.

The fitness industry has made it seem like movement is really complicated or that it's an all-or-nothing situation (we're looking at you, Nike)! Movement is natural. We all can and should do it!

Strength

The key to making your muscles stronger is working them against resistance, whether from lifting weights or using gravity like in yoga. Beauty lies in strength! We like to think of strength training as longevity training. In fact, resistance training is the best way to get rid of fat.

A pound of muscle weighs exactly the same as a pound of fat, but the muscle is denser, so it takes up less space. And so will you!

Further, a pound of muscle burns three times as many calories as a pound of fat.

> *Myth: My muscle has turned to fat.*
>
> *Truth: Not possible! Your fat can increase over time as your muscles decrease from lack of exercise, but they are two different types of tissue. One cannot turn into the other.*

Testosterone is the hormone that is most helpful in promoting protein synthesis (i.e. building strong, shapely muscles). Men make this is their adrenals and testes. But women make it too (in their adrenals and ovaries). To make more testosterone, do more strength training. It's the absolute opposite of a vicious cycle!

Endurance

Endurance refers to the ability of the body's circulatory and respiratory systems to supply power during physical activity. To strengthen the heart muscle and improve its efficiency, try activities that keep your heart rate elevated at a safe level for a sustained length of time like walking, swimming, or bicycling. The activity you choose does not have to be overly strenuous to improve the endurance of your heart and lungs. In fact, over-exertion places your body in a catabolic state, where cells are dying off more quickly than they are being replenished. Start slowly with an activity you enjoy, and gradually work up to a more intense pace. But keep challenging yourself.

If it doesn't challenge you, it doesn't change you!

Flexibility

Flexibility is the range of motion around a joint. Good flexibility in the joints can help prevent injuries through all stages of life, allowing us our independence as we age. Without sufficient stretching, adults lose up to 30% of their flexibility between the ages of 30 and 70. Why does this occur? There are several reasons. By the time people reach their late 20s, they have already lost 15% of the body's moisture content in the muscles. This is why the older people get, the more often they experience muscle strains and sprains. Muscle fibers start to adhere to one another, preventing those fibers from gliding smoothly against each other as our bodies move. Over time, this creates scar tissue. Stretching is a healthy movement pattern that stimulates the production of tissue lubricants, so that muscle glide occurs without resistance.

When we stretch, one muscle contracts while the other lengthens. In yoga, we strive for a balance between support and movement. Yoga poses rely on both static stretching and isometric toning. In many muscle-building poses, the muscle strains against the resistance of our body weight, but the length of the muscle doesn't change. This helps to build strong muscles without creating muscles so pumped up that it limits our range of motion.

Muscle is actually an incredibly regenerative tissue. Your skeletal muscle cells, under healthy conditions, don't undergo cell division. However, they're sprinkled with small satellite cells throughout the tissue. When a muscle is injured, the immune system "cleans up" the site of the injury and those satellite cells get to work. But each time a muscle heals itself, it also leaves behind scar tissue, which creates further tightness and increases the opportunity for injury.

Always attempt to stretch without compromising the integrity of the tendons and ligaments. Tendons are white, avascular tissues that connect bones to muscle. They grow out of the connective tissue of one bone, continue growing through and around the muscle, and then attach to the end of another bone. Ligaments connect bone to bone inside the joint capsule.

Muscles can contract to one-half their resting length and can stretch to double their resting length. Muscles have more elasticity than collagenous structures like tendons, ligaments, and fascia. When a muscle is stretched, it will return to its original length without consistent stretching. When we overstretch tendons and ligaments, they remain too long, resulting in destabilized joints. Tendons and ligaments will take a 6-10% increase in length before they tear. Connective tissues (like tendons, ligaments, and fascia) can take between 1-7 years to heal properly. Erin tore her hamstring tendon in gymnastics when she was 16 and there remains instability at that site to this day!

We in the yoga world are starting to see many injuries from overstretching. Why do you think this is? One reason is that that we are constantly learning new things about how muscles and connective tissues respond to stretching.

If you were under general anesthesia, you would have complete and even excessive range of motion! That means we could lift your leg and touch it to your nose, no matter how "tight" your hamstring is in your waking life!

So why do muscles give resistance when we stretch them? It's because our nervous system is trying to protect us. Let's say you're standing up and try to bend over and touch your toes, but your hamstrings won't let you put your hands on the floor. It's really your nervous system saying it doesn't feel safe going further. So what to do?

1. Stay mindful and remember to breathe. Calming the nervous system will soften the muscle and connective tissue and allow you to stretch safely.

2. Strengthen your core. So often, we are too weak in our core muscles. So the muscles around the core like the pecs, deltoids, traps, hamstrings, or

quads act like an emergency brake in a car to hold everything together.

3. Stretch more often. Your body takes the shape you place it in most often. So if you sit hunched over a computer for 8 hours a day, your body will adopt that basic shape (hunched shoulders, forward head, really tight in the back of your body and too weak in the front). A day filled with various functional movement patterns is the healthiest choice.

If you want to improve your flexibility, try activities that lengthen the muscles like yoga or pilates. But moderation is key. Deep, intense stretching is counter-productive as our joints require some stability that overstretching can compromise. That's why our yoga classes emphasize strength and stability over stretching.

Mind-Body Connection

Staying mindful as you move helps you become more mindful in all areas of your life. For novice meditators, it's often easier to become aware of your body as it moves compared to when you're being still. When we're sitting still in meditation, the sensations that arise in the body are very subtle and harder to discern to than those that arise while we're moving.

The mind can also be very influential on exercise performance. Through the use of visualization, meditation, and positive affirmations, people are able to vastly improve their athletic goals.

How Much Should I Move? Follow the Four!

Each week, you should perform each of these four activities.

1. Yoga
2. Resistance Training

3. Woggle or Walk
4. Something That You Love

1

Yoga

Yoga is for everybody and every body. You don't have to be flexible, strong, young, or beautiful to practice yoga. You don't have to wear expensive clothing. You don't need to become a vegetarian. Maybe you're feeling nervous or insecure because Facebook and Instagram idolize these lithe, beautiful yoginis in these seemingly unattainable poses. Yes, they are beautiful. But so are you!

If you can breathe, you can do yoga!

We get really frustrated when a stranger says that they'd like to do yoga but they can't because they aren't flexible. Being flexible isn't a prerequisite for practicing yoga, though it's a lovely by-product. There is a collective perception about yoga that, we believe, is a little slanted. Social media has been responsible for postulating this idea of what makes a "real yogi". We now equate yoga with Lululemon and juice detoxes and giving up meat or bread. Yoga means wearable mala beads, chanting and little statues of Ganesh. We think real yogis are beautiful and thin, and float around in a state of bliss, drunk on deep breaths and deep backbends. And while some of this is true some of the time, to believe it all is utter rubbish.

Real yogis are carnivores, vegans, and anything in between. Real yogis have temper tantrums and bad hair days and lie awake at night worrying about the mortgage. Real yogis tell fibs and drink too many cocktails and steal pens from work. Real yogis lose their jobs, lose their spouses, and lose their minds occasionally. Real yogis catch colds, get cancer, and even die. Real yogis are everyday people trying to make a little more sense of this crazy world by expanding their consciousness.

Yoga isn't ultimately about standing on your head or touching your toes. It's about learning how to connect to the moment rather than run from it. It aims to help us quiet our monkey minds, if only for a moment, from a judgmental, reactive mind. It allows us to simply be. If you can breathe, then you're a real yogi. Like the Velveteen Rabbit, if you have the capacity to love and be loved, then you're real.

And that makes you a yogi.

> **Journal Prompt**: What does yoga mean to you? Which of the truths or untruths are preventing you from trying?

Erin's Edition:

Run, Erin, Run!

One of the greatest pleasures of my life is working with private clients after surgeries like hip or knee replacements. I have students with heart disease, cancer, and autoimmune disorders. Some of my clients have bunions or scoliosis or COPD. And they are all simply beautiful when they're on the mat. Getting to witness anyone aligning his or her body, mind, and breath is beautiful.

I was born severely pigeon toed. A well-respected orthopedic surgeon told my parents I would never run and probably always walk with a limp. As soon as I started walking, I was fitted for metal leg braces. Remember those white baby shoes parents would have bronzed in the 70s? Now picture those shoes with metal rods running up from the inner and outer foot to the top of the thigh, where they attached with Velcro. There was a metal hinge at the knee that allowed me to bend my knee just a tiny bit.

The rods forced my feet and legs to point outward, in an attempt to change the shape of my skeleton as I grew. I don't remember being fitted for the braces, as I was only three, but I completely believe my parents when they say that I hated those things. They slowed me down. All toddlers have an agenda to explore as much of the world as they can before nap time and I was no different. I would get frustrated with the braces and shake my legs in the vain hope that they would just fall off.

My parents thought the "never run" diagnosis was a little harsh to hang on a three-year-old. So they enrolled me in dance and gymnastics and a yoga class taught at our local co-op. During these classes, I got to take my leg braces off and just move my body like all the other kids. Again, I don't remember any of this. But there are pictures of me in these classes and the jubilant smile on my face says it all. I fell in love with moving my body in all kinds of ways. I wasn't especially graceful or skilled. I fell off the balance beam, forgot my dance choreography, and toppled in my tree poses. But I laughed and begged to go back, week after week.

Movement became my haven, a place where my mind would shut

down and I could get lost. It was just me and the barre or the vault or the mat. Me and the music, some sweat and my breath. And I truly believe these classes acted as physical therapy, allowing me to far surpass the expectations of my orthopedist (I don't limp even a little). As I got older, I tried it all. Cheerleading, karate, running, dancing, weight-lifting, aerobics, swimming, surfing, and woggling.

Movement has been the longest and truest love of my life. It is in my DNA and yoga is my first and truest love. Yoga gives us the physical benefits but so much more. Yoga teaches us to be present with uncomfortable sensations and experiences.

Let's say you move into triangle pose and want to get out. Your hamstring is tight. Your core is being challenged. Your mind wants to be anywhere but here. But you don't give up. You settle in. You hang there, present, noticing the thoughts and sensations as they arise. This helps us deal with the ups and downs of life off the mat as well. Yoga and mindfulness go hand in hand. Time on your mat will often fulfill your Invite, Move, and Rest intentions for the day (and twists are so good for your digestive system, we'll throw in that Digest intention as well). Listen to your breath and mindfully move in a way that supports your overall intention for the day.

A Quick Anatomy Lesson

If I peeled off your belly skin (uh, gross), there would be a layer of fat. If I scraped away the fat, the first layer of muscle is the rectus abdominus (that "6 pack" that women's magazines get so worked up about). The oblique muscles form a "V" under that, running from the side ribs down to your pubic bone. Under the rectus and obliques lies the transverse abdominus, the deepest of the abdominal muscle layers. It runs horizontally from your lower ribs to your pubis and acts like a girdle, wrapping around your body. Did you know you cannot even wiggle your fingers without your transverse abdominus contracting? So learning to use it intelligently builds core stability. We also consider your psoas (hip flexor), glutes, and the muscles that run along the spine to be core muscles.

So how to use them without overusing them? In almost every pose, draw the front ribs slightly into the body (think about the bottom of your breastbone "kissing" the heart). This is your solar plexus, your energetic center of raw power and control.

Engaging the Core

Yoga teachers throw this phrase about hither and yon, but what in the hell does it actually mean? We want you to learn to move your body from a strong, stable core all the time, on or off the mat.

There are two types of muscle fibers in the body: white, fast-twitch muscles and red, slow-twitch muscles (to distinguish between them, think of white lightning and a red stop sign).

Core muscles have more red, slow-twitch fibers. If we can train them to provide stability and support, we can relax the white, faster-twitching muscle fibers. This is a releasing of chronically tight muscles. Over engaging those white, fast-twitch muscles creates tension. They are supposed to be used for short bursts of energy, but we overuse them, asking them to hold our skeleton up indefinitely. They get tired easily, so they then recruit surrounding soft tissues, resulting in stiff joints and overly tense muscles in the hips, neck, and shoulders.

If we train the red, slow-twitch muscles to engage, our core gets a constant flow of blood (this is where the red comes in) and creates a strong, supported body where we can actually let go of the tension in our necks, shoulders, and hips. Red, slow-twitch fibers have so much blood flow that they repair and rebuild tiny tears in the fibers more quickly, allowing us to train them every day.

The Practice

We often think about how our daily life activities are like a prison cell for our joints. Too much sitting, too much driving, and too much stress really locks our spine down, limiting our range of motion.

> *Myth: I'm not burning enough calories in yoga.*
>
> *Truth: First, the calories. If you are mindfully eating real food, you don't need to be counting calories. Remember, all calories are not created equally so fill your body with the good ones and leave out the CRAP. Now to the yoga! We wonder if those perpetuating this myth have ever really done a yoga class. There are as many different forms of yoga as there are kinds of body types. Different classes focus on differing aspects of stretching, strengthening, breathing, etc. but there is a class for everybody. Just like any other fitness class, a good yoga class incorporates many aspects of movement, but a bonus with yoga is the mind-body connection often lacking in basic fitness classes. It's these layers of a yoga class that distinguish it from other types of exercise. You might have to try a few before you find your preference, but no one I know would say that yoga doesn't burn calories. That's just ridiculous!*

The **Jellyfish Flow** is your "Get Out of Jail Free" card! Practice this one every day to say hello to sweet freedom in your body. You could do the whole thing in five minutes without sweating, so no excuses about how you don't have time!

Want to turn up the heat? Add on one, two, or all three **Fiery Sun Flow**

sequences.

Feeling more introspective? Skip the sun flows and go directly to the **Cooling Moon Flow**.

Once you're warm and loose and in your fabulous flow state, practice one or both of the **Floor Flow** sequences. **Spicy Floor Flow** focuses on gaining muscular strength, where **Cooling Floor Flow** focuses on gaining muscular length.

Roll down onto your back for the **Core Power Flow**. Then add on one or both of the **Gentle Back Flow** series. Let those stretches be long and juicy and delicious.

Finally, **Shavasana** is a must with every single practice, no matter how long or short. Have you ever been super-stressed trying to get to a yoga class? A late babysitter or too much traffic means you arrive harried and frazzled. But 90 minutes later, you float out of the room without a care in the world. Much of this bliss is due to shavasana.

Shavasana is that crucial time where our energetic body can absorb the work of the poses. Quieting the mind creates this deeply restful place where the body can heal itself, growing stronger and healthier each time.

Basically, you should aim to do the **Jellyfish Flow** and **Shavasana** (or another restorative pose) every day. Mix and match the other sequences based on your physical, mental, and energetic needs. The endless combinations keep it interesting.

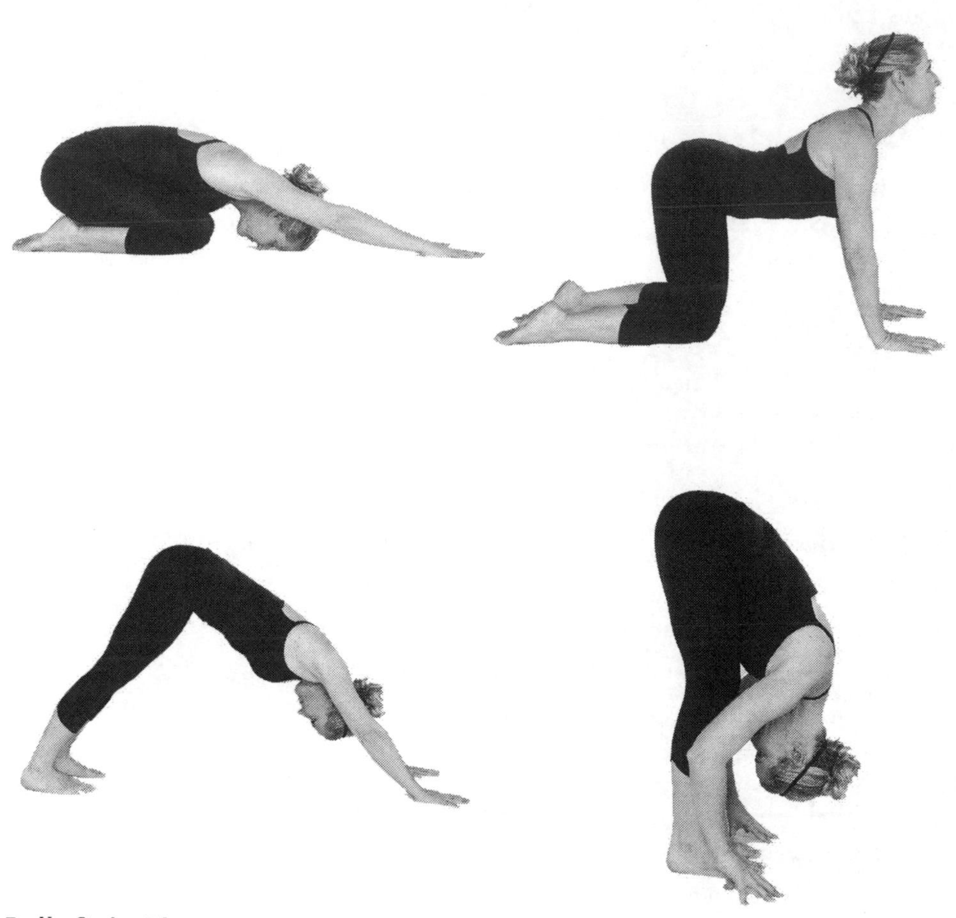

Jellyfish Flow

1. Start in **child's pose.** From all fours, draw the hips back to rest on the heels, leaving the arms extended to stretch the shoulders. You can widen the knees here or place a blanket under the knees if it feels more comfortable. Close your eyes. Start to engage the ujjayi (ooh-JAY-ee) breath. With the lips pressed together, say "AH" as you inhale and "HA" as you exhale. Imagine you are

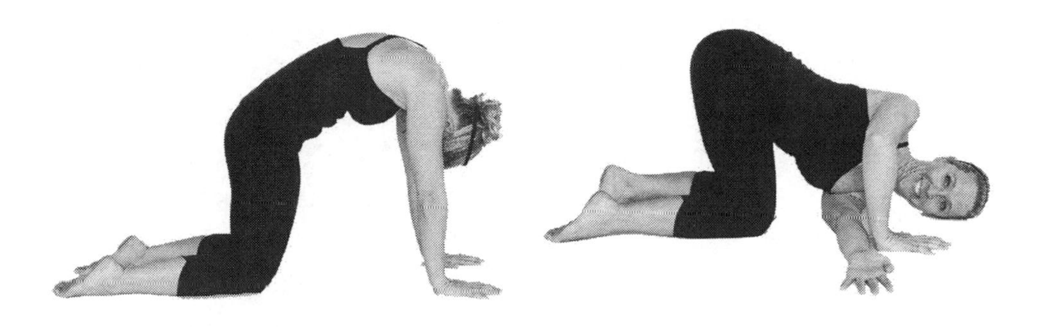

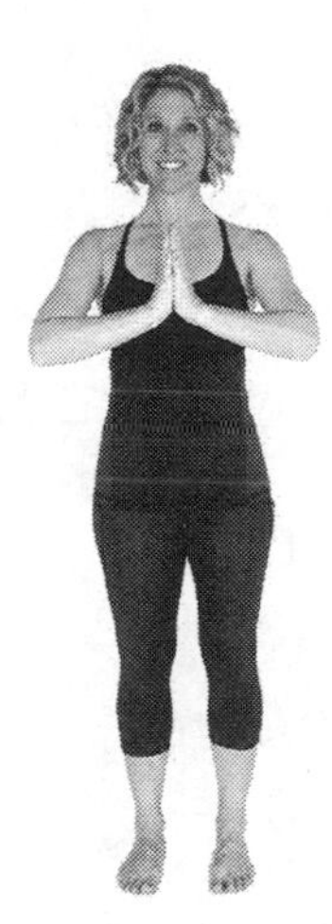

fogging a mirror in the back of your throat - keep the breath soft and relaxed. It sounds like Darth Vader a bit, or like when you hold a conch shell up to your ear. This breath opens the lungs a bit more and focuses the mind.

2. From child's pose, rise up to tabletop. Stack your shoulders over your wrists and your hips over your knees. Draw the front ribs slightly into the body, feeling the back of the heart rise toward the ceiling. As you inhale, drop the belly toward the floor as the tail and the head both lift, moving into a back-

bend (**cow pose**). Exhale and tuck the chin and tail as the spine rounds toward the ceiling (**cat pose**). Do this 5-15 times, imagining each breath loosening the muscles on either side of your spine.

3. Return to tabletop. Take the left arm and reach it under the right arm as the left side of the head comes to the floor. Rest the left shoulder on the floor as well, looking up over the right shoulder into **tangled cat**. Hold for 5 breaths and then switch sides.

4. Return to tabletop. Spread the fingers evenly so that the middle fingers are parallel. Now walk the hands one hand-length forward, so they are slightly in front of your shoulders. Curl your toes under and lift your hips to the sky to form an upside down "V" as you move into **down dog**. "Walk the Dog" to wake up the hips and legs by bending one knee and then switching. Then press both heels toward the earth and your thighs toward the back of the room. Imagine someone is pulling a rope around your thighs to the back of the room, internally rotating the thighs a bit. The tailbone reaches slightly toward your heels to protect the lower back and hamstring tendons. Draw the front ribs slightly into the body, feeling the shoulder blades draw around a little toward your heart. The head hangs heavy and relaxed. Hold 5 breaths.

5. From down dog, lift the gaze toward the hands and then step the feet forward to the top of your mat into **uttanasana** (**standing forward bend**). The feet are parallel to each other and the knees are slightly bent. Let the spine and head just hang here and enjoy the stretch in the back of the body. Hold for 5 breaths.

6. Bending the knees more, tuck the chin and slowly roll up to standing in **mountain pose**. From the side view, your ears are stacked over your shoulders and your hips over your heels. The crown of the head lifts toward the sky so that the back of your skull is parallel to the wall

behind you. Hands rest at heart center in **anjali mudra**. A mudra is a yoga pose for your hands. Anjali Mudra (hands at the heart) is a symbol of gratitude. Shoulders are relaxed down the back. The floating ribs pull slightly into the body, as does the navel. The feet are parallel to each other. Breathe deeply here for 5 breaths before moving on.

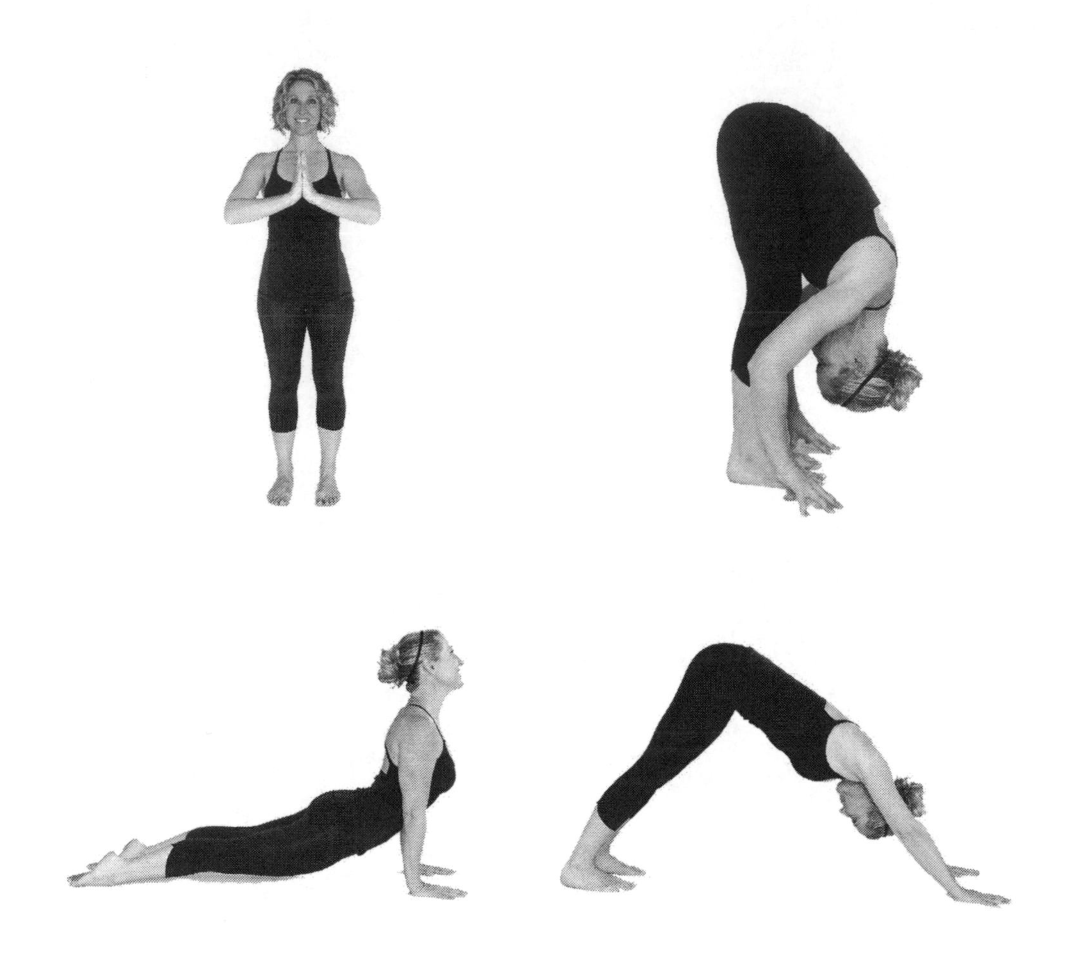

Fiery Flow 1

1. From **mountain**, fold over into **uttanasana**.

2. Step the feet back into **plank pose**. Imagine you are in a horizontal mountain pose. The shoulders are stacked over the wrists like in tabletop, but the legs are straight. Never lock your elbows. There is a soft bend in the elbows so you are using your arm muscles to hold you up (rather than your elbow ligaments). To

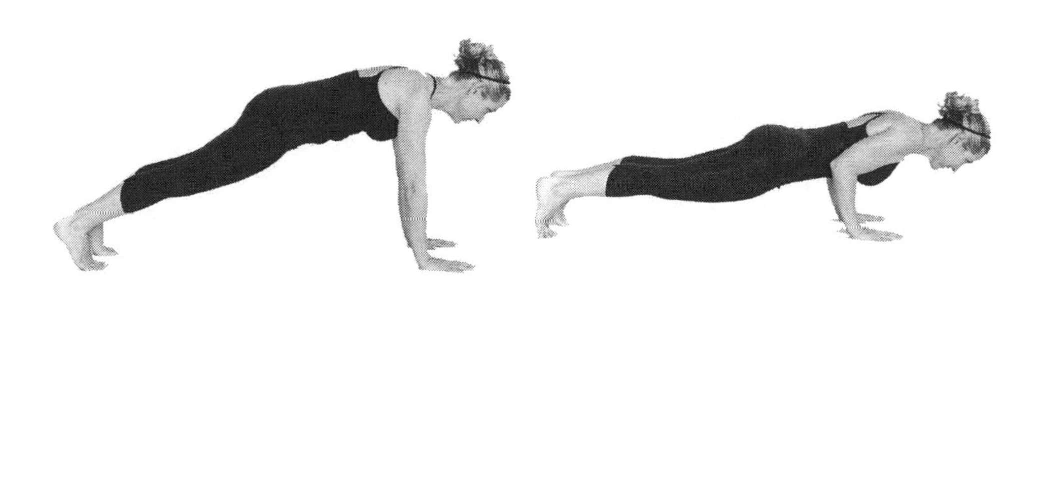

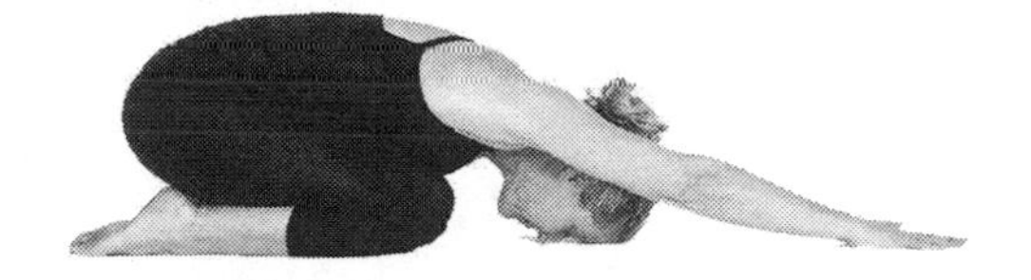

engage the core, your spine will actually be in a little tiny cat pose here so the upper back is flat or slightly rounded (there shouldn't be a "valley" between the shoulder blades). Don't let the low back fall toward the floor - rock that solar plexus strength! Engage your thigh muscles and press the heels toward the back wall so your booty doesn't lift too high. Lift the chin a little off your chest and feel your collar bones get wide. Hold here for 10 strong breaths.

3. Inhale and shift the shoulders forward over the fingertips. Exhale and low-

er halfway to the floor in **chaturanga** (the "yoga push up"). Your elbows will graze the sides of your ribs. Never let the shoulders drop lower than the elbows. Keep the upper arms parallel to the floor or even the shoulders slightly higher. Engage that core!

4. Now, one at a time, press the tops of the feet into the floor. Press the arms straight and lift the chest and legs into **up dog**. The eye of your elbow faces forward, but don't lock the elbows. The thigh muscles are strong here. Look straight forward or slightly up, but don't throw the head back too much. Try to lift through the side ribs. The corners of the mouth turn upward. This is the perfect time for a grin!

5. From up dog, curl the toes under (one foot at a time). Pull the solar plexus in as strongly as possible to lift you back to **down dog**. You can press to table then to down dog if you prefer.

6. Rest in **child's pose** for 10 breaths before moving on.

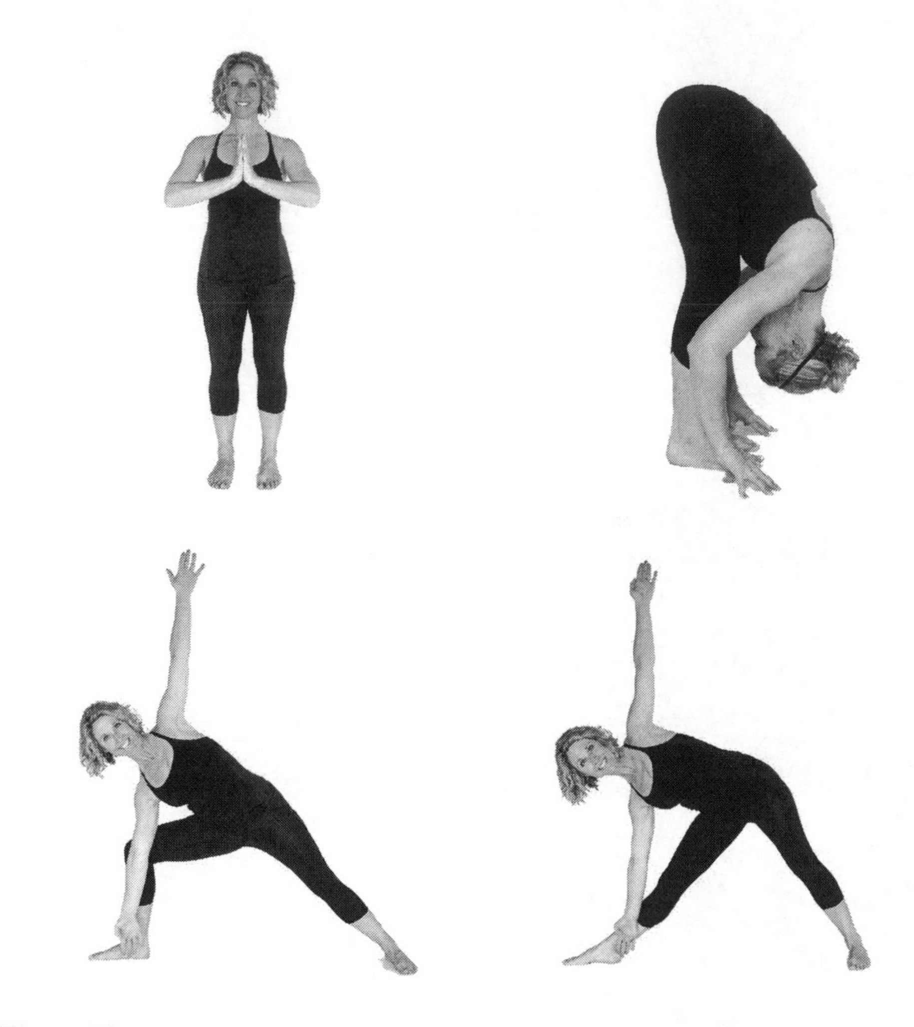

Fiery Flow 2

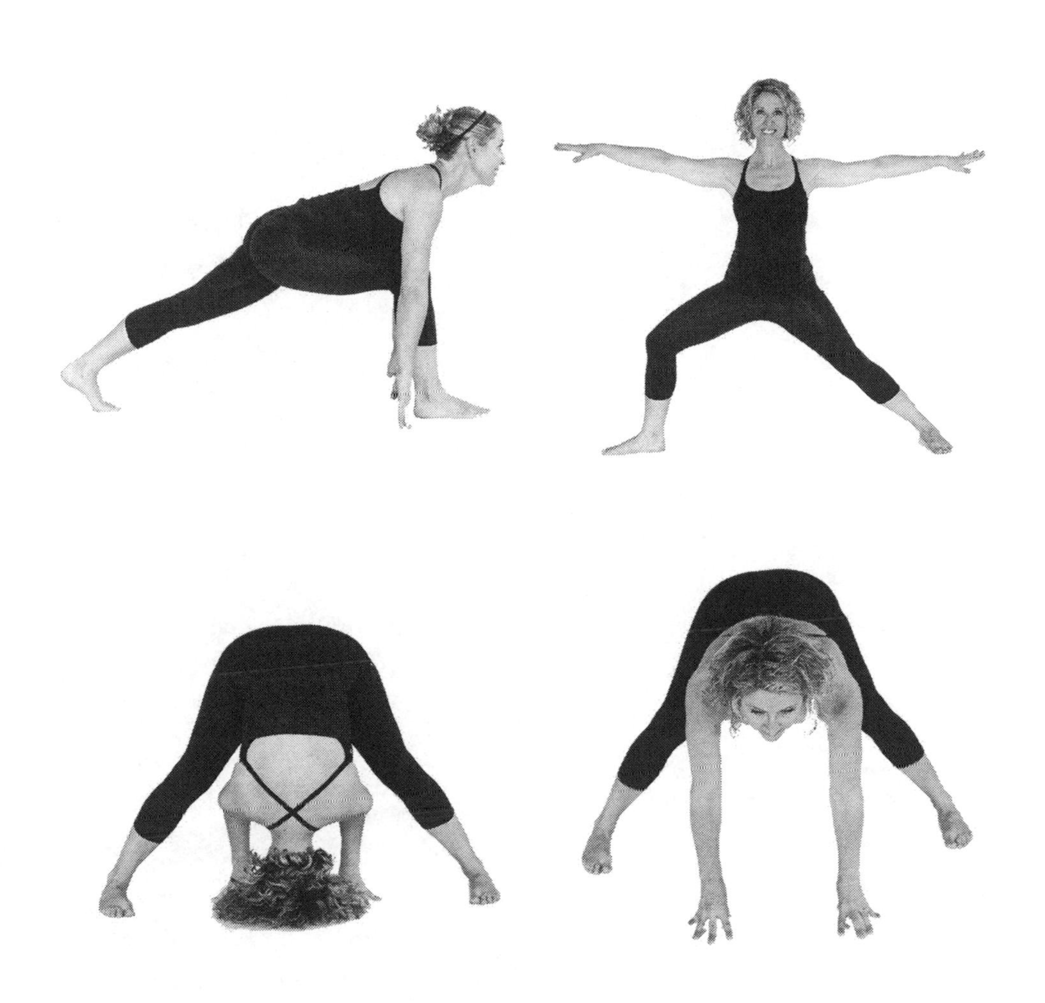

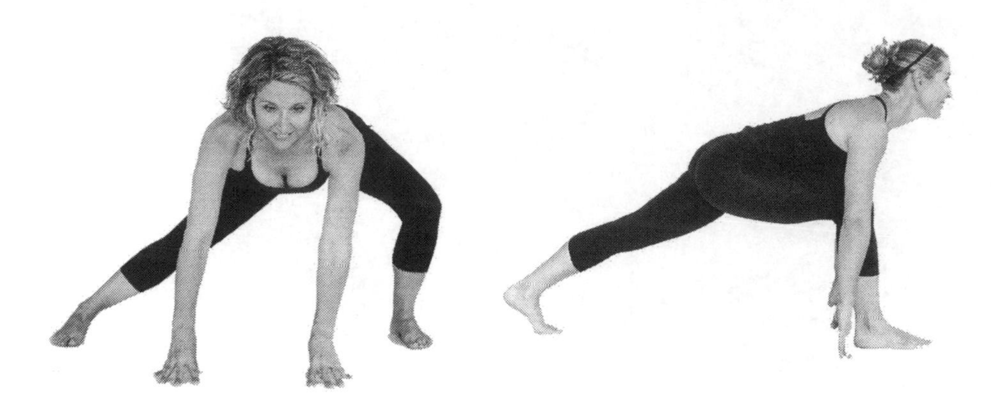

Fiery Flow 2 (continued)

1. From **mountain**, fold over into **uttanasana**. From here, step the left foot back into **up runner pose**. The right knee will be bent 90 degrees and sit right over the ankle. The left leg will be strong and stable. The fingertips are resting on the floor under the shoulders, framing the heel.

2. Now "warrior prep" the back foot, spinning the toes out and dropping the heel to the floor. The toes of your back foot will point to the top left corner of your mat. As you root your feet into the floor, lift your torso up to face the left side of the room. Arms reach out in a "T." The front knee stays right over that ankle (if you peek down, you should be able to see the big toe of your front foot). This is **Warrior II**. Bring to mind a warrior. How do they look? Feel? Act? Bring these strong, fierce qualities to your pose. The limbs are strongly engaged and the heart is wide and open. Find your fierce here for 5 breaths.

3. Leave the lower body as it is. But tip forward at the waist now and place your right forearm on your right thigh. Stretch the left arm overhead at a diag-

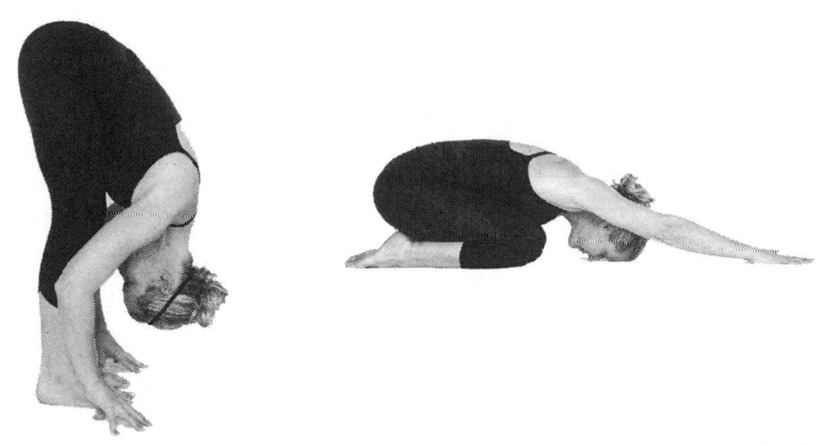

onal, palm facing the earth into **extended angle pose**. Imagine your body is being squeezed here between two panes of glass, pulling the right booty cheek underneath you as you roll the left hip up and back. Keep spinning your heart to the left and slightly upward. Breathe deeply for 5 breaths.

4. On an exhale, start to straighten the front leg into **triangle pose**. Bend the front knee as much as you need to keep an appropriate (as in not too much) stretch in your hamstring. The right hand can rest on the shin, ankle, or on a block. The left arm reaches high into the air.

5. Now turn both feet to face the long left edge of your mat and fold over into **standing straddle**. The feet are parallel to each other and the head and spine are hanging. Let go here and breathe deeply. Let gravity work its magic on the spine and let your thoughts fall away. Shift your awareness here from the breath into that space that floats between each breath. Hover in the place of stillness. Let your intuition decide when it's time to move on.

6. When it feels right, place the hands under the shoulders and lift your chest. Bend the left knee, pressing the knee slightly toward the left with-

out turning the foot out. Enjoy that stretch in the right inner thigh. When you're so moved, switch sides. We call this a **Water Warrior**. Move fluidly between the two a few times.

7. Now turn to the front of the room and frame the hands around the right foot as you return to **up runner** pose. Step forward into **uttanasana** and repeat the sequence with the left foot forward.

8. Rest in **child's pose** for 10 breaths before moving on.

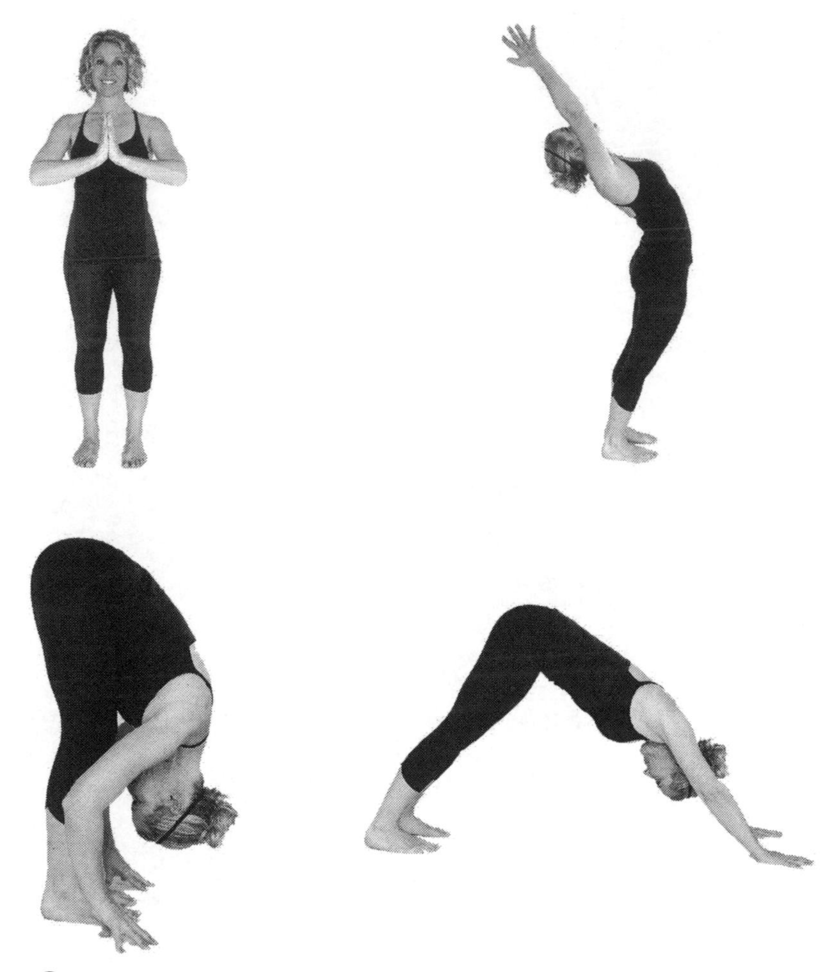

Fiery Flow 3

1. From **mountain pose**, swing your arms out and up, bringing the hands together overhead as you look toward your thumbs. Gently lift your heart to lean back into **upward mountain** (a standing backbend). Be mindful not to throw the head back too far. If you notice you're holding your breath here, it's probably because you're leaning back too far.

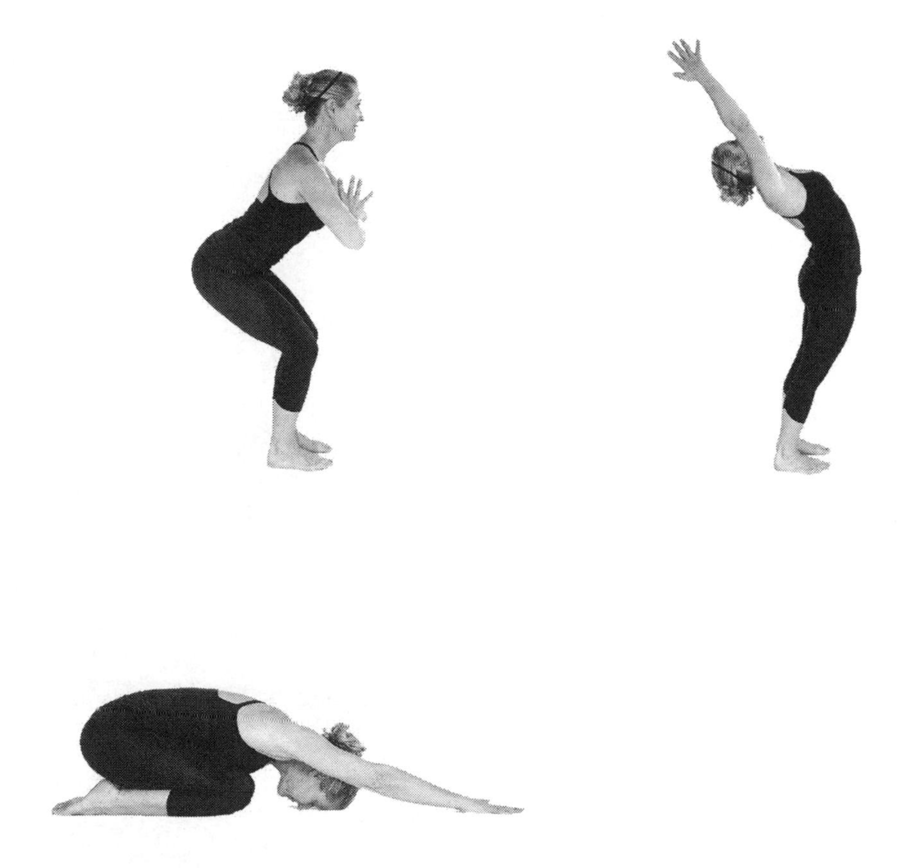

2. As you exhale, sit down into **chair pose**, bringing the hands to the heart in **anjali mudra**. Feet and legs are parallel to each other and the knees are stacked over the ankles (not the feet). Imagine you're going to tap your booty down on a barstool.

3. Moving with the breath, repeat this flow sequence (**upward mountain to chair pose**) 15 times. Remember that every time you bring your hands into anjali mudra, you are saying "thank you" to the Universe.

4. Then fold over into **uttanasana**. Step back into **down dog** and rest in **child's pose**.

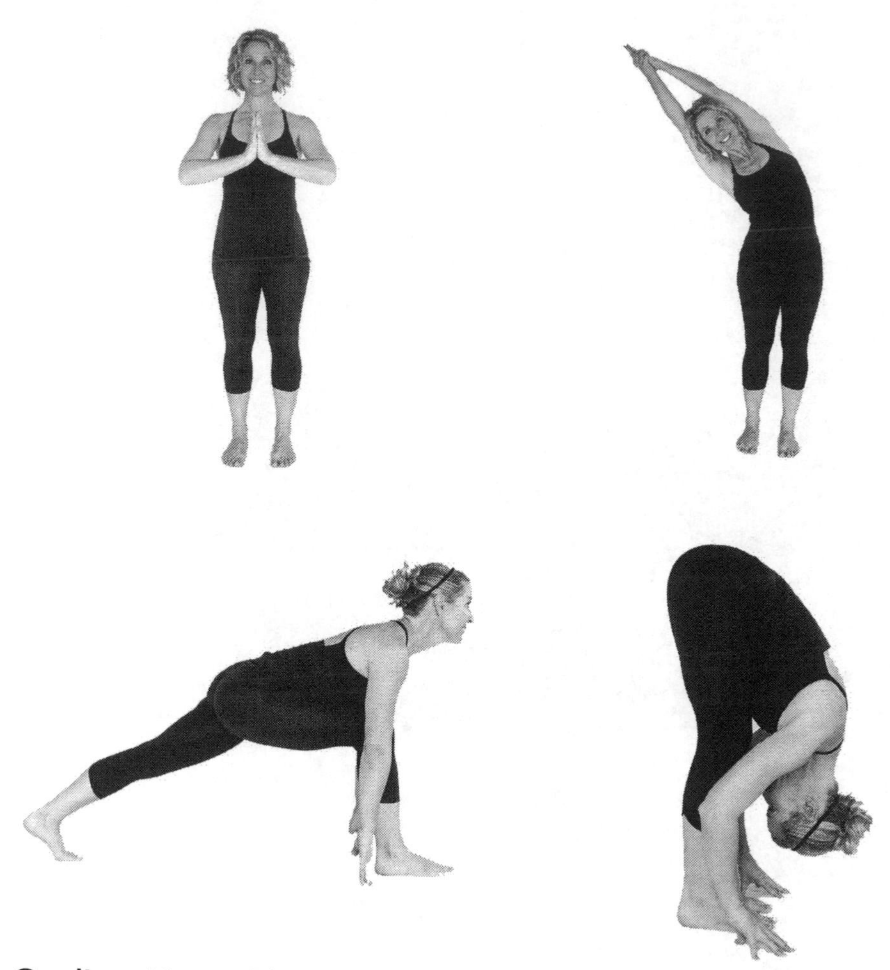

Cooling Moon Flow

1. From **mountain pose**, extend the arms over head and bring the hands to touch. Keep the chin parallel to the floor and the gaze on a horizontal plane. Tip like the proverbial teapot to the right, rooting down firmly with the left foot into **standing side stretch**. Hold 3 breaths and then switch sides.

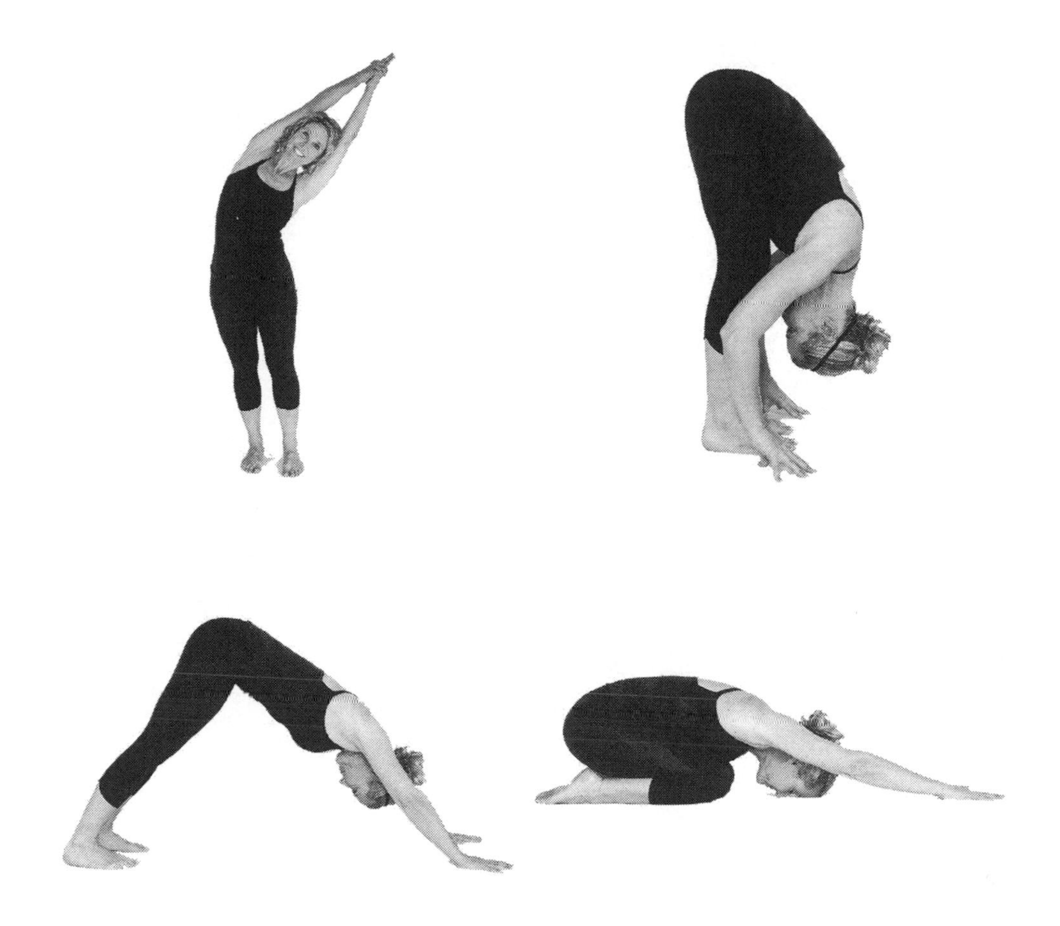

2. Fold over into **uttanasana**. Step the left foot to the back of the mat into right **up runner**. Gently bring the left knee to the floor (use a blanket under the knee if necessary) and lean into **low lunge**, reaching the arms up by the ears.

3. Curl the left toes under and step forward into **uttanasana**. Repeat **low lunge** on the other side.

4. Lift the hips, stepping your right foot back to meet the left in **downward dog**.

5. Rest in **child's pose** for 10 breaths before moving on.

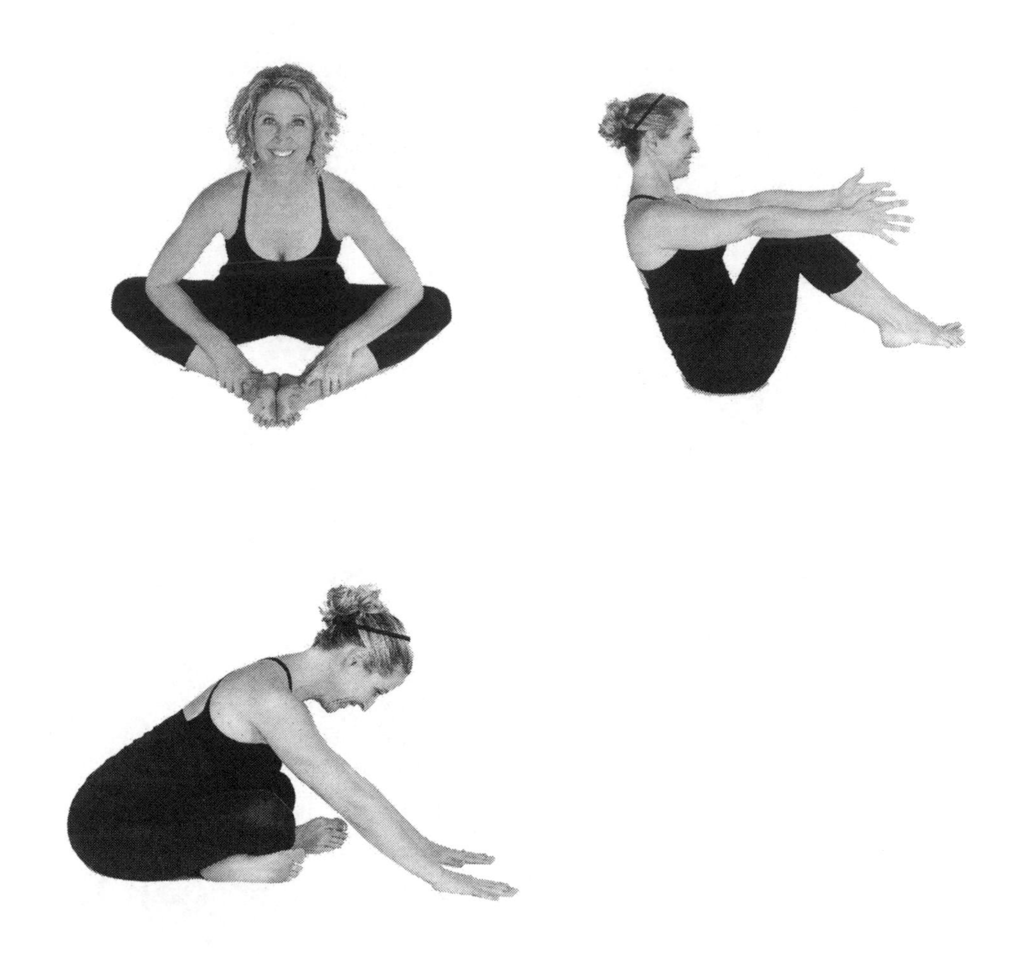

Spicy Floor Flow

1. Come to sitting on your booty with the bottoms of the feet together. Hold the ankles and lean forward, trying to keep the spine long. This is **baddha konasana**, the cobbler's pose. Imagine you're a cobbler trying to see the soles of your shoes. Enjoy a lovely stretch in the hips and thighs for a few breaths.

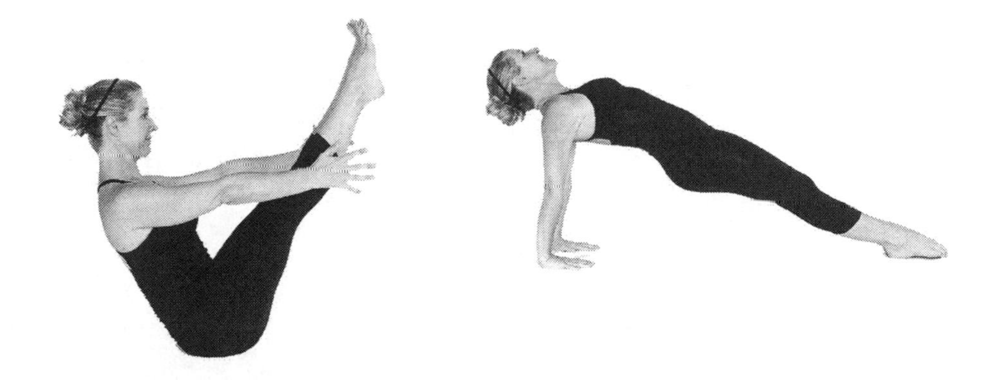

2. Lift the knees together and raise the toes off the floor as the arms reach long, parallel to the floor, in **boat pose**. Connect to a strong solar plexus (reread the section above about engaging the core) here for 10 breaths. Really turn up the volume by straightening the legs!

3. Extend the legs long on the floor and sit up tall. Place the hands behind you, just under or slightly past the shoulders, fingers facing toward your booty. Inhale and lift your heart and hips to the sky. Try to press the bot-

toms of the feet to the floor as the body lifts. Chin can stay tucked to the chest or, if it feels OK in your neck, the head can drop back to stretch your throat. This is **purvottanasana** (**eastern stretch**).

4. As you exhale, release the booty to the floor and fold over your legs into **paschimottanasana** (**western stretch**). Hands can just rest on the floor wherever they feel able, but keep the spine long and the collarbones reaching towards your ankles.

5. Moving with the breath, repeat this flow sequence (**purvottanasana to paschimottanasana**) 10 times. Yoga was traditionally practiced facing the sun (that's where the yoga term "sun salutes" comes from). Since the sun rises in the east, the front of our body is referred to as the "eastern side" and the back as the "western side" in the yoga tradition. So lifting the heart stretches the "eastern" side and folding forward stretches the "western" side. Get it?

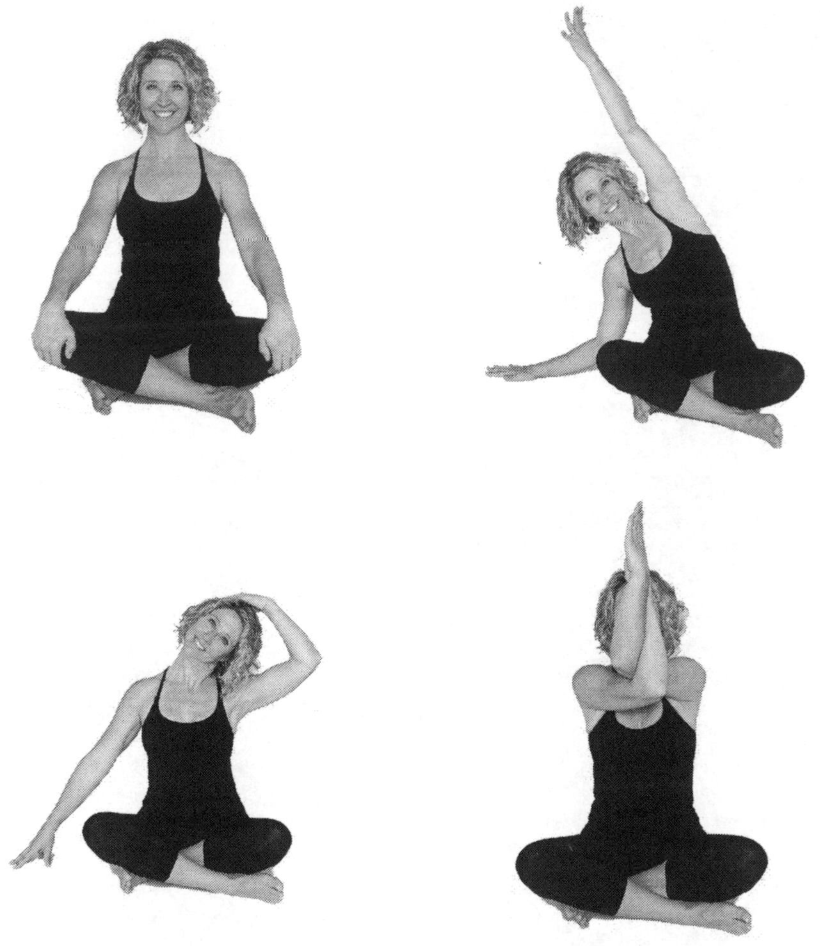

Cooling Floor Flow

1. Sit cross-legged, flexing the feet to protect your knees. Fold forward and linger here in this blissful hip release. When the spirit moves you, switch sides and repeat **cross-leg fold** on the other side.

2. Sit cross-legged and bend to one side, resting one hand (or elbow) on the

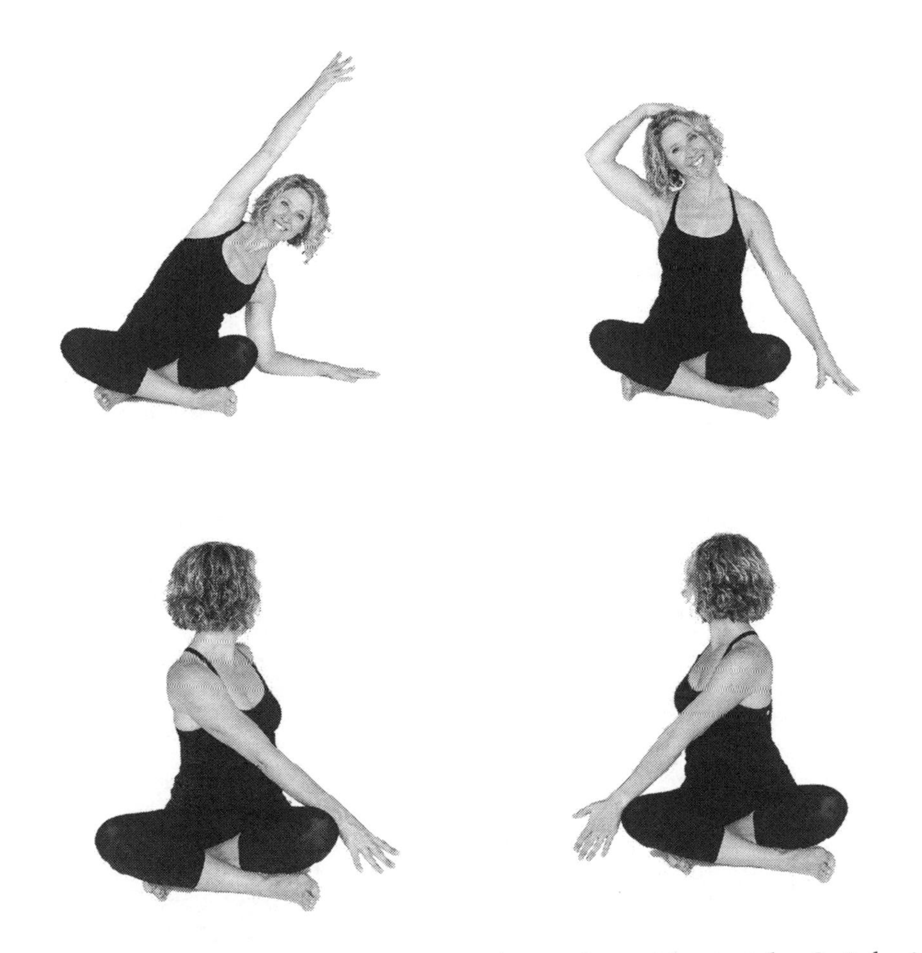

floor as the other arm reaches up and over for a **side stretch**. Switch sides.

3. Sit back up tall. Drop one ear to the shoulder. Let the hand gently guide the head down as the other arm "walks" out away from the body into a delicious **neck stretch**. Do both sides. Hunching over a phone, computer, or steering wheel takes a toll on our necks. This is the remedy! Linger and loiter here, really reveling in the sweet release of that neck tension.

4. Cross one elbow on top of the other and twist your forearms up like ivy climbing a vine into **head of the cow arms**. Attempt to bring the palms to touching, spinning the thumbs back towards your face. Lift the elbows up and press the forearms forward, parallel to the front wall. It feels delightful to shake the head "no" here. Make sure to switch sides.

5. Finally, place the left hand on your right knee. Place the right hand on the floor behind you. Breathing in, sit up really tall. Breathe out and twist your heart towards the right, looking over your right shoulder into **seated twist**. Hold 5 breaths and then repeat on the other side.

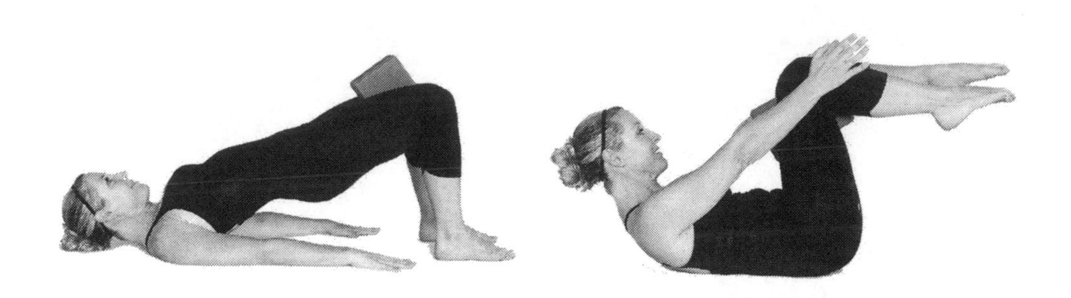

Core Power Flow (you'll need a yoga block)

1. Lie on your back with your knees bent, feet flat on the floor and legs parallel to each other. Place a yoga block between your thighs and start to gently squeeze the inner thigh muscles around the block. Lift your hips off the floor until you form a straight diagonal line from your shoulders to your hips in **bridge pose**. This is the "in" breath.

2. As you breathe out, lower the hips and draw the knees in toward the chest, peeling the shoulder blades off the floor as you raise your chest and reach your fingers toward your heels in the **egg pose**. Keep squeezing the tissues of your inner thighs around that block!

3. Moving with the breath, repeat this flow sequence (**bridge to egg with block squeeze**) 20 times.

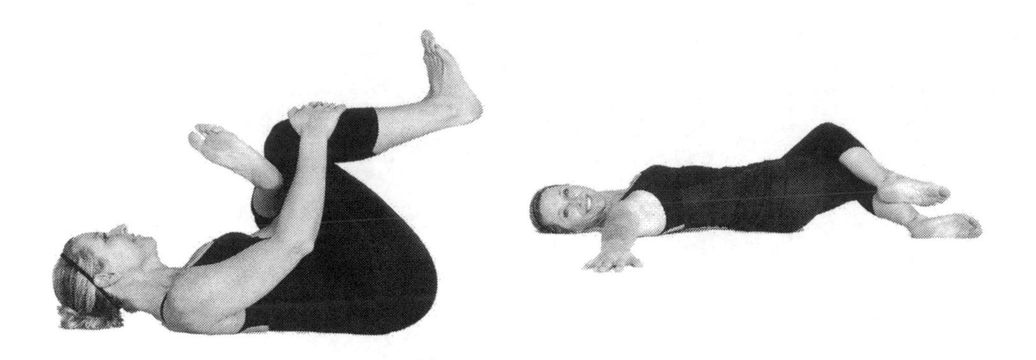

Gentle Back Flow 1

1. Yay! We finally get to lie down! The Yoga Gods were looking out for us when they gave us hip openers. They feel wonderful, so stay in each one as long as you'd like. Lie on your back with your legs bent, feet flat on the floor. Place the right ankle on your left thigh (just above the knee), flexing the right foot to protect your knee ligaments. Now lift the left foot off the floor, hugging the left thigh in towards your chest into **sleeping pigeon pose**. Gently press the tailbone towards the floor. The hip and thigh stretch is intense but so tasty! This one's great for sciatica.

2. Now cross the right thigh over your left thigh. Imagine you have on a robe without any underwear - that's how you want to cross the legs here. Drop your arms into a "T" and let the legs fall with gravity to the right for a **back and waist stretch** of the left side.

3. Lift the legs up and shift your hips to the right a smidge. Now drop your arms into a "T" and let the legs fall with gravity to the left for **lying twist**. Look to the right, trying to roll the ribcage to the right as the hips keep spiraling to the left.

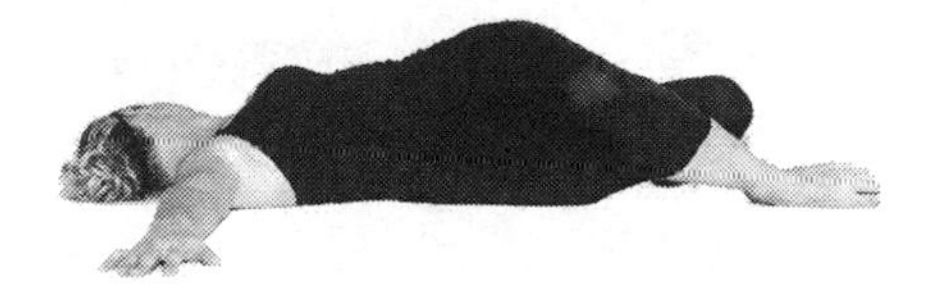

4. When you feel ready, repeat the whole series on the other side.

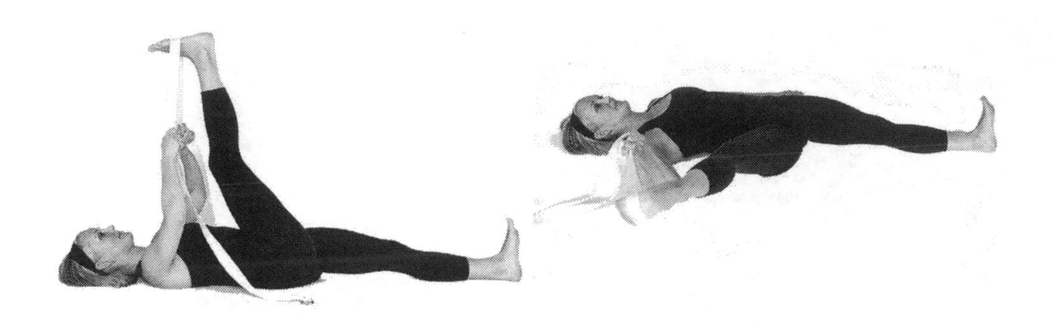

Gentle Back Flow 2 (you'll need a strap)

1. Stay in each of these poses as long as you'd like. Place a strap across the ball of the right foot. Extend the left leg long on the floor and start to draw the right thigh toward your belly for **lying hamstring stretch**, holding the strap with both hands. Keep the left foot straight or slightly turning inwards. The left thigh should press down to the floor. The right leg will eventually be perpendicular to the floor. It's fine to keep a little bend in your right knee here. As long as you keep your hips and back releasing into the floor, you won't strain your lower back (which happens sometimes in standing hamstring stretches).

2. Hold the strap with the right hand only. Keep the left side of the body (ribs, booty, and hip) rooted down as you drop the right leg out toward the right. The right foot moves up toward the shoulder a bit (without lifting the left pelvis off the floor or losing the position of the left leg).

3. Lift the right leg back up and switch the strap into the left hand. Draw the leg across the body to a 45° angle. Now try to draw the right hip back down towards

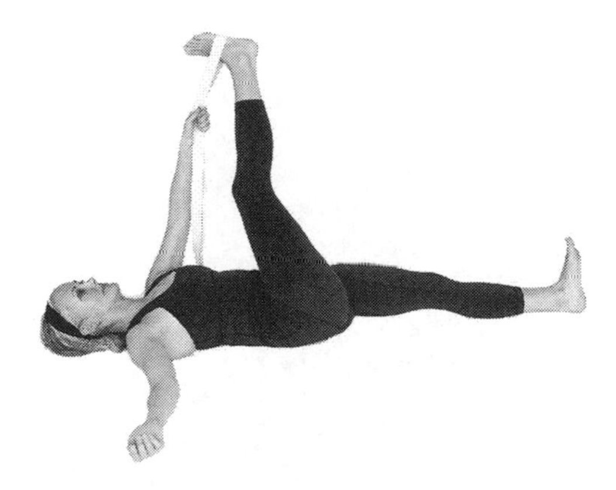

the floor (yowza, right?!) The foot can move slightly towards the back wall.

4. When you feel ready, repeat the whole series on the other side.

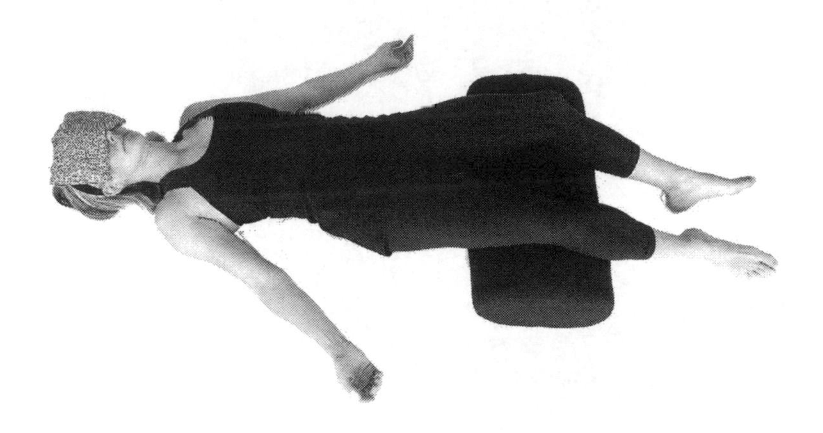

Shavasana

Think of your body as a battery. If the poses are where you're using electricity and heat, then shavasana is where you're recharging.

Using your smart phone, record yourself reading this section. Then, for the first few times, play it back as you follow the directions. Once you get the hang of it, you'll be able to easily find this yummy place by yourself.

Lie on your back with a bolster under your knees to release your lower back. Separate your feet about eight to ten inches apart. Turn the palms upward to relax the shoulders - the fingers will curl in as if you're holding a ball of warm light. Place an eyebag over your eyes. We always get cold, so we like to place a blanket over our feet. Fidget until the physical body is really comfortable. Now take a really, really deep breath in and open your mouth to audibly sigh it out. As you hear that exhale, feel the body melting into the floor. Starting at your toes, mentally scan up through your body, pausing to become aware of each area and to release any tension you notice. Soften the belly and notice how it lifts and lowers with the breath. Release any tension in your jaw, so the top and bottom teeth fall away from each other. Let the eyes drop back in the skull. Smooth the skin on your forehead.

Notice any thoughts now. When you become aware of a thought, plan, or worry, simply let it go. Shift your awareness to the breath. Breathe in and be aware that you are breathing in. Breathe out and be aware that you are breathing out. Then shift the awareness from the breath to the tiny little space that lies between each breath. In yoga, this is called the kumbaka. You aren't creating the pause – it's already there. You're just being more mindful of it. Let the inhale come naturally, filling the belly. Then hover in that stillness before the body feels it's time to exhale. At the tail end of the exhalation, float in the pause there as well.

Remain here several minutes, being cautious not to drift off to sleep. When you're ready to come out, start to lengthen your inhales. Then gently wiggle your fingers and toes. Rock your head from side to side. Stretch your arms overhead. Take a really noisy yawn. Roll over onto your right side and rest here for a minute. Use your left hand to lift yourself up to a seated position.

Sit in cross-legged pose with the hands in anjali mudra, the hand seal symbolizing gratitude. Take a few breaths. Thank your mind, breath, and body for the myriad ways they support you every single moment of your life. ***Namaste***.

To access yoga videos with Erin and Andra, visit www.theOMplace.net.

2

Resistance Training

Almost weekly, women tell us they don't want to lift weights because they don't want to get big muscles. But unless they are injecting testosterone (which we highly discourage), this is impossible! Because of testosterone levels, male and female bodies respond differently to exercise. Both get stronger, developing appropriate musculature while also strengthening ligaments, tendons and bones.

But women simply do not produce grotesquely large muscles because of lower testosterone levels. Women do, however, produce the exact musculature needed to keep their bodies lean, their bones strong, and their ligaments and tendons functioning well.

> *Myth: I walk or run, so I don't need to do other kinds of exercise.*
>
> *Truth: Walking or running is great, but those activities should be coupled with other strengthening and stretching exercises. Think exercise diversity and move your body in as many ways as possible a few days each week. If you are just doing one type of exercise, then you are just strengthening your muscles and bones in one way. You want to incorporate movement that strengthens all parts of your body. This is how you stay strong as you age. This will also help to keep exercise interesting and fun!*

OK, time for a little good news, bad news. Let's get the bad news over with first. Starting in our 30s, we lose a half pound of muscle every year if we are not strength training. That's an average of five pounds every decade! If you are not making muscles, the ones you have are atrophying and your body composition is changing. When your body composition changes, that means the muscle is decreasing and the fat is increasing. That's why people become weaker and flabbier as they get older. This has become an accepted progression in our society but it does not have to be this way!

We should not view aging as becoming weaker and flabbier with an "oh, well" kind of attitude. When your body becomes weak and out of shape, you are more susceptible to injuries in your joints. Have you ever heard someone say they can't workout because they have a bad back? In most cases, they have a bad back because they don't work out and their core muscles are simply weak! In addition to bodily injuries, decreased muscles and increased body fat means you are more susceptible to lifestyle diseases like hypertension, diabetes, obesity, cardiovascular diseases, and cancer.

Remember when we said that lifestyle diseases account for more deaths world-wide than infectious diseases for the first time in history? It's all the more frustrating because it is entirely preventable. These injuries and lifestyle diseases can be combated to a significant degree by simply changing the muscle composition of your body, eating a diet of real food rich in nutrients and low in processed foods, and managing your rest and stress levels.

Age affects our resting metabolic rate. We stop growing bone after the age of 25, so the metabolic rate goes down by 2 percent or more per decade after that. Further, as we near perimenopause and menopause, our bodies make less and less estrogen, resulting in a slower metabolism. This means we burn about 50 fewer calories per day. But we can turn back that infernal clock by vowing to never diet again!

Our bodies will make sure they get what they need to function. If the body can't get it from nourishing, nutrient-rich food, it will break down our muscles to keep the body running.

But here's the good news: a basic schedule of resistance exercise that targets all the major muscle groups in your body 2-3 times per week is the most effective counter to muscle loss. All people can begin to build muscle, no matter their age or current physical state. Strength training is the process of exercising with progressively heavier resistance to stimulate muscle development. The primary outcome is stronger muscles and the secondary outcome is stronger tendons, ligaments and bones. It's a win-win!

Sarcopenia

Sarcopenia is muscle loss resulting from inactivity and the natural aging process. Somewhere in our 30s, we stop growing muscles as easily as we did when younger and begin to actually lose muscles if we don't use them. Ever heard the saying "use it or lose it"? Well, we're certain that this is where it originated!

Inactive people in their 30s and older can actually lose 3-5% of their muscle mass per decade. In day-to-day life, muscle loss means a decrease in strength and mobility, while increasing the likely occurrence of injury. In other words, we just can't move around like we used to. Loss of muscle mass also results in higher body fat content, weakened skeletal system and a slower metabolism. None of that really sounds great.

We don't have to accept that this is the natural path of aging. We don't have to accept that our strength, bones and joints will just wither away without us being able to do anything about it. We can do something about it. Use it or lose it!

The primary treatment for sarcopenia is resistance training - exercise that increases strength through the use of resistance like weights and bands. Research has shown that anyone at any age, no matter how much muscle they have lost, can begin to rebuild their muscular and skeletal strength in as little as two weeks! Your body responds so quickly to resistance training because that is exactly what it has been waiting, hoping and praying that you give it!

Andra's Addition:

After becoming a personal trainer and yoga instructor, I naturally believed all my family members had floppy cores and needed to build themselves some muscle! At my request, my husband Travis and I began a progressive 3-day-a-week pushup challenge. I love old-school pushups because they strengthen a common weakness, can be executed quickly, don't cost anything and are always available. Pushups can be a satisfying place to begin resistance training, because results come quickly if you do them regularly and this can foster a motivation to build more strength, something we both really needed!

Three weeks in, we were gaining strength and increasing our pushup numbers well but, to my shock and surprise, Travis had surpassed me at an alarming rate. He could pump out those pushups with seemingly little effort and in rapid succession, easily doubling and tripling my numbers. What was happening?

Well, testosterone was happening. Testosterone is a male sex hormone pretty much responsible for everything that's amazing (and not so amazing) about men. Although men produce and need more testosterone than women, testosterone production is important for women as well.

Generated in the ovaries and adrenal glands, testosterone production in women is less than a tenth of that of men. Despite this small amount, recent research shows that low testosterone in pre and postmenopausal women can affect sexual activity, lean body mass, energy level and a general sense of happiness. Until recently, the focus on the "female" hormones progesterone and estrogen overshadowed testosterone in women's health but it is becoming clear that testosterone isn't just for men!

However, this topic is somewhat controversial. We are not recommending testosterone or hormone supplements of any kind. Nobody except your own body knows how much testosterone you need. As should be clear from our Digest section, we believe in acquiring things our bodies need from the most natural source possible. You are surely asking, "how does one acquire testosterone from the most natural source possible?" Well, the answer is Resistance Exercise! That's right - grab your weights and leave the prescription at the doctor's office!

Many studies show that resistance exercise increases testosterone production in men and a few studies show that it does in women, but that's OK because it's just common sense! When we lift weights regularly, our testosterone and other hormones begin to regulate themselves to proper levels. In fact, our entire body begins to regulate itself to proper levels. That's why everything about your body and your mind feels better when you start making muscles regularly.

Your body not only wants to lift weights, it was designed and has evolved to lift, push, and pull, thereby generating muscles! No matter your gender, age or physical condition, your body is praying to the Higher Power that you will get up and start making more muscles. If you listen, here's what you'll notice:

- Increased interest in sex (who doesn't want that?)
- Lower body fat and higher muscle mass leading to a faster metabolism
- Enhanced overall body strength, flexibility, and balance
- Strong bones to fight osteoporosis
- Improved joint strength
- Higher energy levels and stamina
- Soothing sleep
- Greater productivity
- Lower blood pressure
- Sharper mind
- Decreased risk of developing cardiovascular disease
- Healthier immune system and therefore fewer illnesses
- Augmented confidence
- General contentment and happiness
- Decreased risk of cancer and diabetes
- Increased ability to handle stress
- A more youthful looking you

Given all that, how can you not want to make some muscles?

Andra's Addition:

A word of caution to women training with a male partner, please don't compare your progress to that of your male partner's (or anyone else for that matter).

Remember Travis and the pushups race? Because of increased levels of testosterone, he'll beat me every time. But that's OK. It's not about me beating him (even though I am really competitive and love to win), it's about both of us increasing our strength and reaping the benefits of that glorious list! Besides, I'll beat him at something else!

Weight Resistance Exercises

Required Equipment:

1. Body Sport Heavy Resistance Double Loop Tubing with 3 pads, Red (available on Amazon.com for about $14.00)
2. SPRI Sponge Ball (available on Amazon.com for about $15.50)
3. Dumb Bells (buy only what you need - we recommend starting with 8-10 lbs)

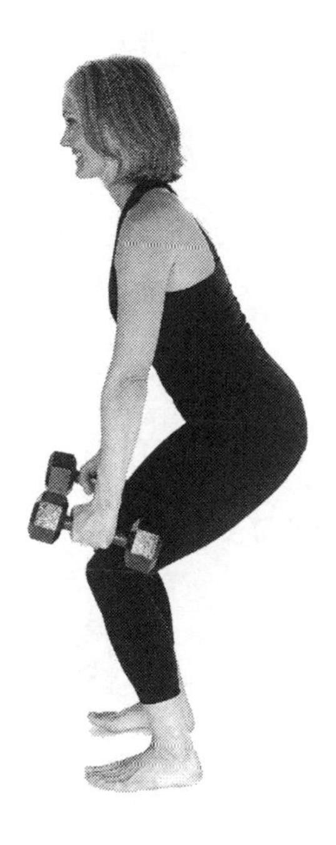

Basic Squat with Dumb Bells

3x10 (That means 3 sets of 10 squats, resting about 30-60 seconds between sets).

With weights in your hands and feet hip width apart, pull your belly in and tuck your tailbone toward the ground. Bend your knees, shifting your hips back but keeping your knees directly over your ankles. If you glance down, you should be able to see your toes, but the weight is in your heels. Engage your glutes and stand back up to starting position. That's one squat! Do 3 sets of 10 squats. When you are in the actual squat, imagine you are in a nasty public toilet and you are trying to pee without touching anything!

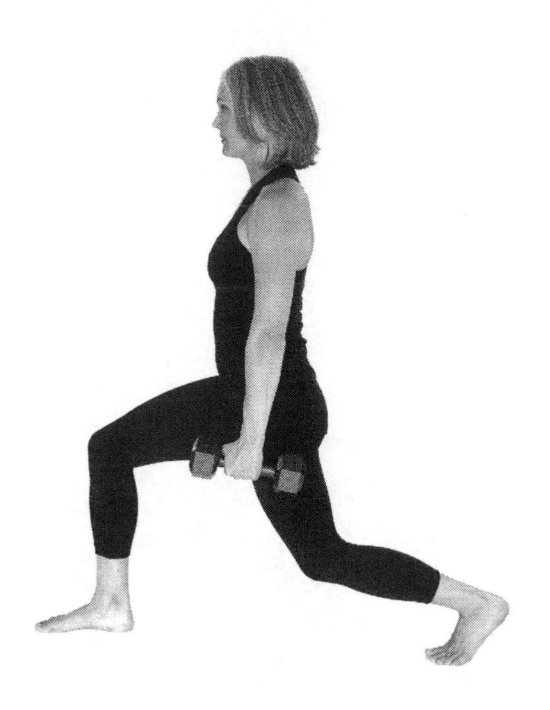

Basic Lunge with Dumb Bells

3x10 (That means 3 sets of 10 squats, resting about 30-60 seconds between sets)

With weights in both hands, step the right foot forward about 2 feet so that you can bend the right knee 90 degrees. Be careful to keep that knee exactly over your ankle, never allowing it to go past the toe. The left knee also bends straight down toward the floor at a 90 degree angle. Lower the back leg down and up 10 times, then switch to the other leg to complete the first set. anything!

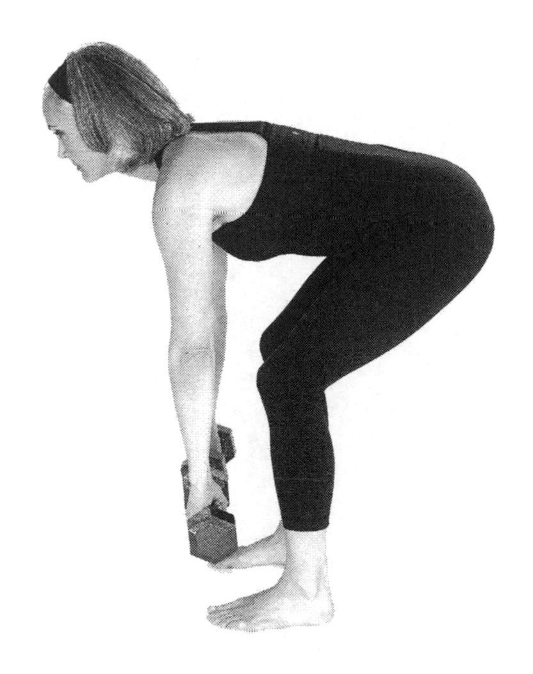

Dumb Bell Dead Lifts

3x10 (That means 3 sets of 10, resting about 30-60 seconds between sets)

Rotate the weights to the front so your palms are facing your thighs. Hinging at the waist, bend forward with a flat back, reaching the weights toward the tops of your feet, but stopping midway between your ankles and knees. Keeping your knees slightly bent and your core pulled in tight, inhale and lift back up to the starting position. It is not a squat where you are thrusting your butt back, but a hinging at the waist with a flat back. Imagine someone being able to serve tea off your back!

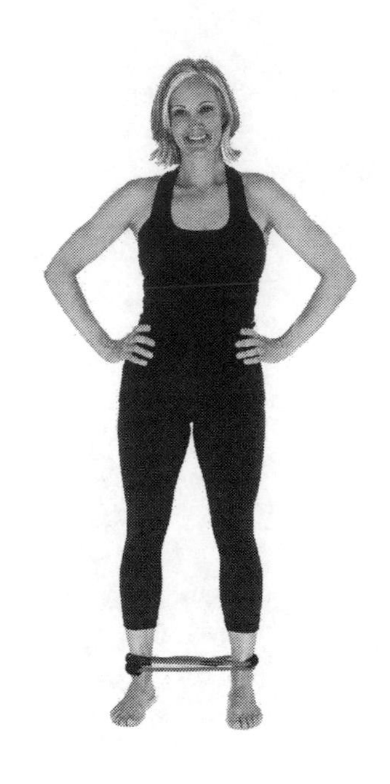

Lateral Crab Walks with Band

3 Times

Find a clear path of at least 25-30 feet (anywhere you can step without running into obstacles). Step through both loops of the Double Loop Band so that both bands are around your ankles. Stand with your feet hip width apart, your left shoulder pointing in the direction of your chosen path. Draw you belly in and tuck your tailbone toward the ground. Step with your left foot pressing as far as you can into the band. Allow the right foot to slide toward the left like a zombie shuffle - remember the work is in the leading left hip. When you reach the end, simply go back to where you started, working the right hip this time. You should feel this exercise strengthening your lateral hips. One set is down your path and back.

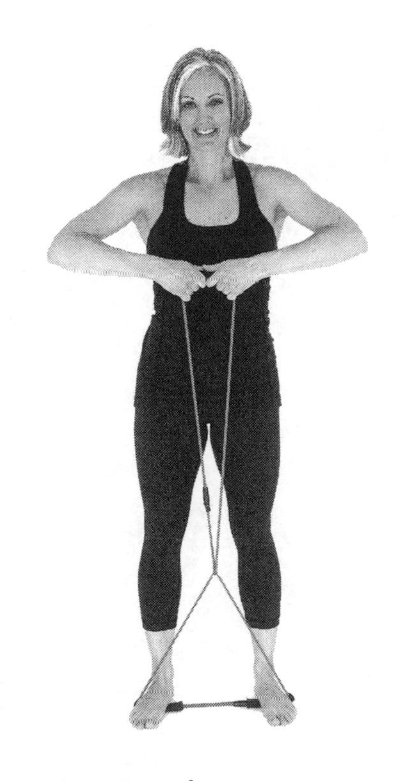

Upright Rows with the Band

3x10 (That means 3 sets of 10, resting about 30-60 seconds between sets)

Taking the loop of the band with the two foam handles, step on the band, placing a foot on each foam handle. Widen the feet to press into the band. Grab the outer edge of the other loop and straighten to a standing position, palms facing thighs. Draw the naval in, to engage the core and lengthen the tailbone toward the ground. Slowly pull the hands in front of the body toward the chest, sending the elbows up and out like bird wings before releasing back to starting position. You should feel this work in the top of your shoulders.

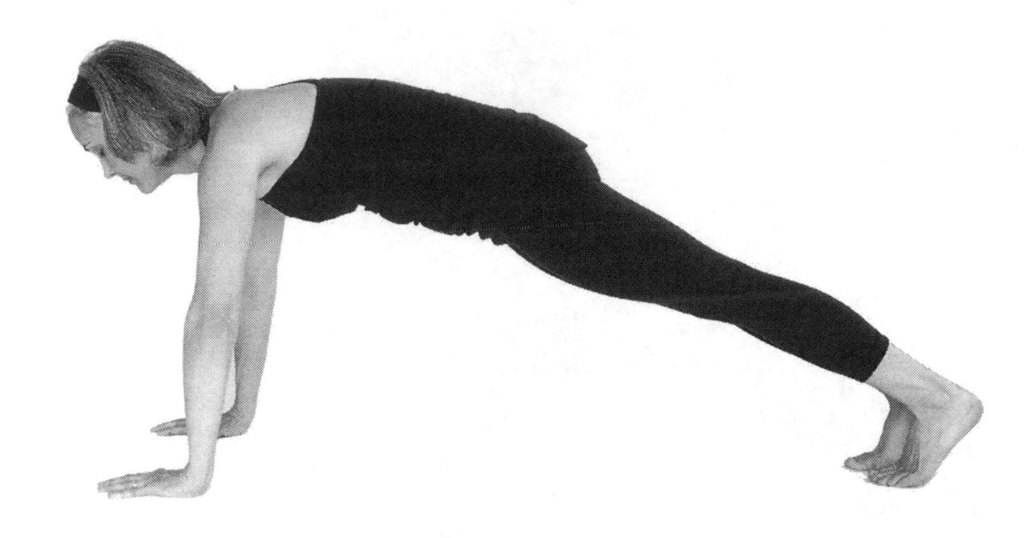

Pushups

3x10 (That means 3 sets of 10, resting about 30-60 seconds between sets)

Do these with straight legs, knees bent, (there's no shame in bent knees - they are still considered pushups) or a combination of the two. Place your palms a bit wider than your shoulders - if you are using a yoga mat, place your hands just outside of your mat on the floor. Shift the weight forward into your shoulders. Pull your belly button into your spine and lengthen your tailbone to point toward your heels. It's exactly the same position if your knees are on the ground. Lower towards the ground, bending your arms 90 degrees. Then press back up to your starting position. Remember that pushups are hard for women because we are usually weaker in our upper bodies, but it's so important to strengthen our shoulders, upper chest and core! Stick with them - they get easier! Andra believes the push-up is the single best exercise we should all do every day!

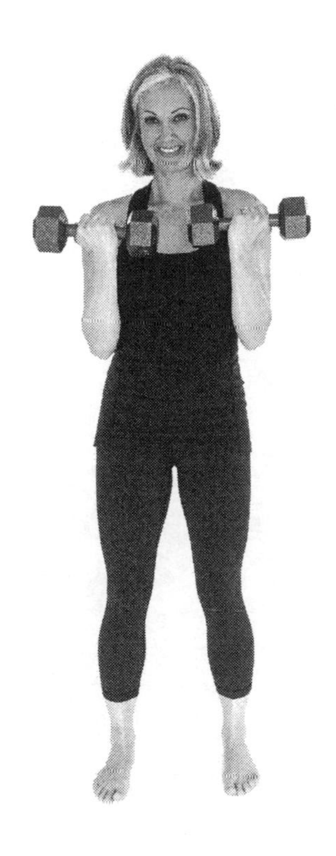

Biceps with Dumb Bells

3x10 (That means 3 sets of 10, resting about 30-60 seconds between sets)

Stand with feet hip width apart while lengthening your tailbone toward the ground. Place a small bend in your knees to protect your lower back. Glue your elbows into your waist, lift the palms of your hands and the weights up toward your shoulders. Pause for a second before you slowly lower them back to the starting position. Keep this movement slow and controlled. Never use momentum - only use muscle power!

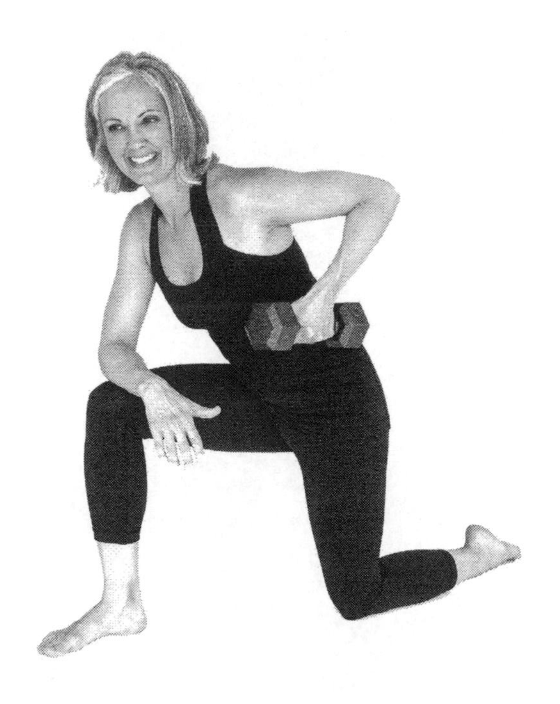

Single One Arm Rows with Dumb Bell

3x10 (That means 3 sets of 10, resting about 30-60 seconds between sets)

Take one weight in your right hand and place your left knee and left hand on a bench, stool, hearth or stable ottoman. Bend over 45 degrees, engage your core, and draw your right arm toward your chest (sending the elbow straight up toward the ceiling). Pause and then slowly and with control, lower back to starting position. Repeat 9 more times before switching to the other arm to complete one set. Do 3 sets of 10 with steady, controlled precision.

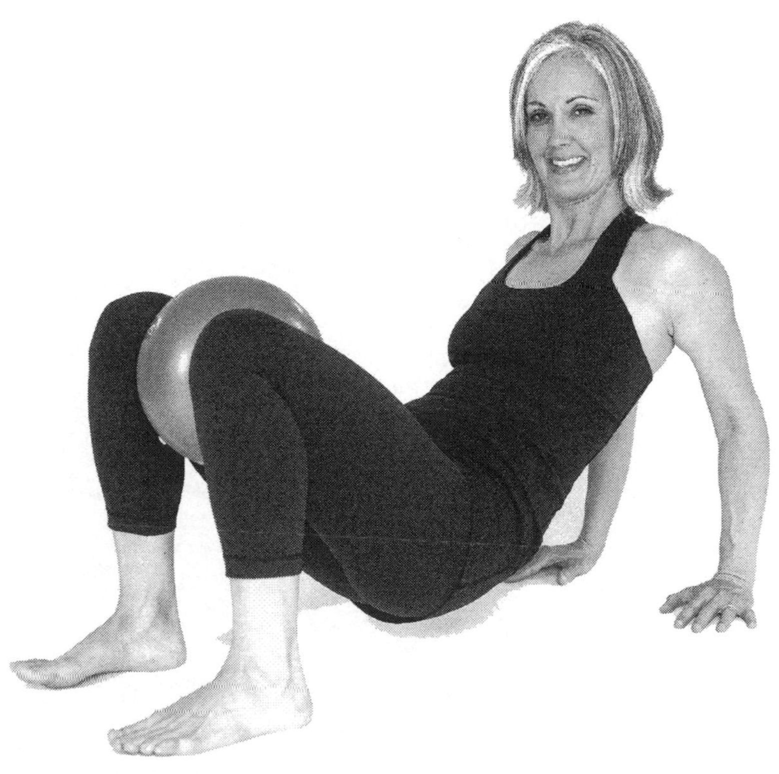

Body Weight Triceps

3x10 (That means 3 sets of 10, resting about 30-60 seconds between sets)

Using a hearth, step, or sturdy bench, sit down on the bench and place your hands on either side of your thighs, solidly gripping the edge. Press into your hands and lift your bottom off the seat. Shift forward so that your bottom can lower in front of the bench. With control, lower your booty, bending only your elbows. This puts the work solidly in the back of your arms (triceps muscle). Squeeze your elbows toward each other, lower slightly down and press back up. This is a very small and controlled movement - think quality over quantity! After 10, lift your bottom back to its original seat and rest for 30-60 seconds before starting the second set.

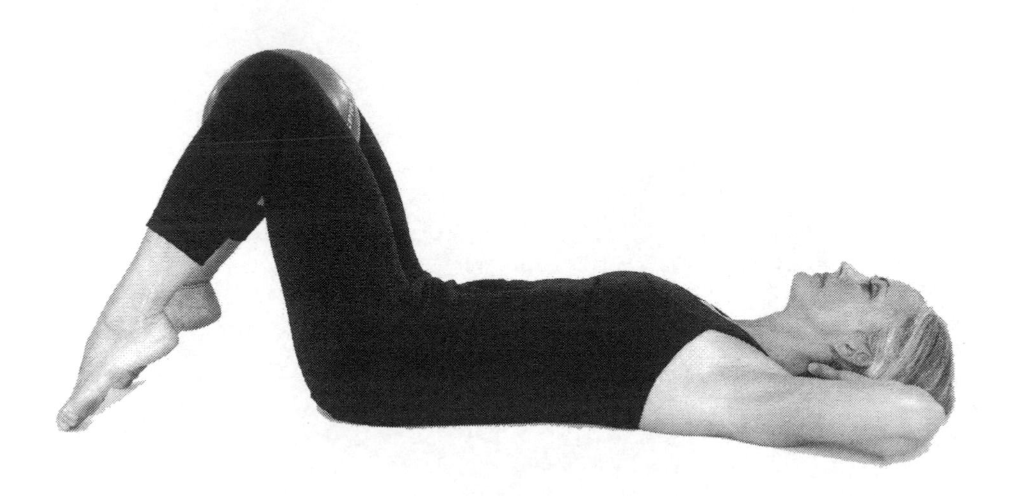

Mindful Toe Taps

3x10 (That means 3 sets of 10, resting about 30-60 seconds between sets)

Lie on your back with your knees bent and your feet on the floor. Place the SPRI Sponge Ball between your inner thighs and gently squeeze. Engage the core, pulling the front ribs down and pressing the back ribs against the floor. Inhale and tap the toes to the floor, all the while keeping the back ribs connected to the earth. Exhale and pull the knees in toward the shoulders, rolling the tailbone off the floor slightly without using momentum. Repeat 9 more times to complete the first set.

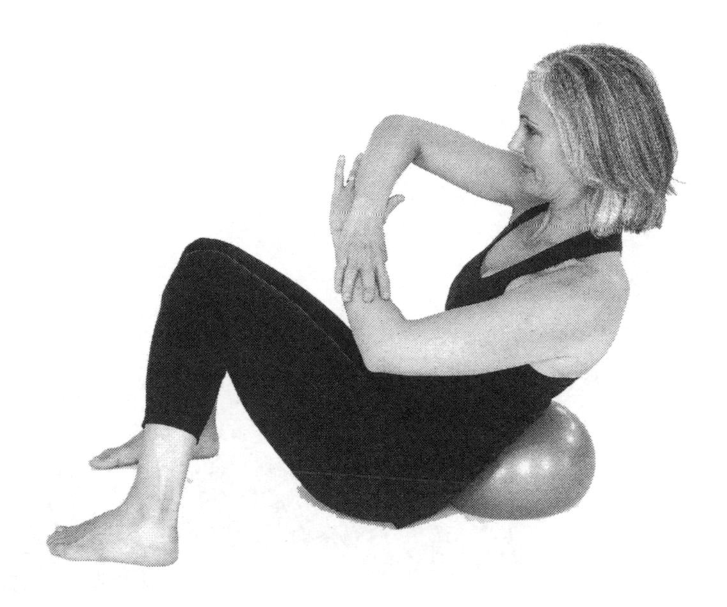

Obliques with SPRI Ball

3x10 (That means 3 sets of 10, resting about 30-60 seconds between sets)

Sit up and place the SPRI Sponge ball behind your tailbone to support your lower back. Bend your knees and draw them together, resting them on one another while the feet spread wider. Stack your hands over one another and extend your elbows out to find your bird wings again. Draw the right elbow to the right hip bone in a small controlled movement, then draw the left elbow to the left hip before returning to the starting position. Repeat 10 times for the first set.

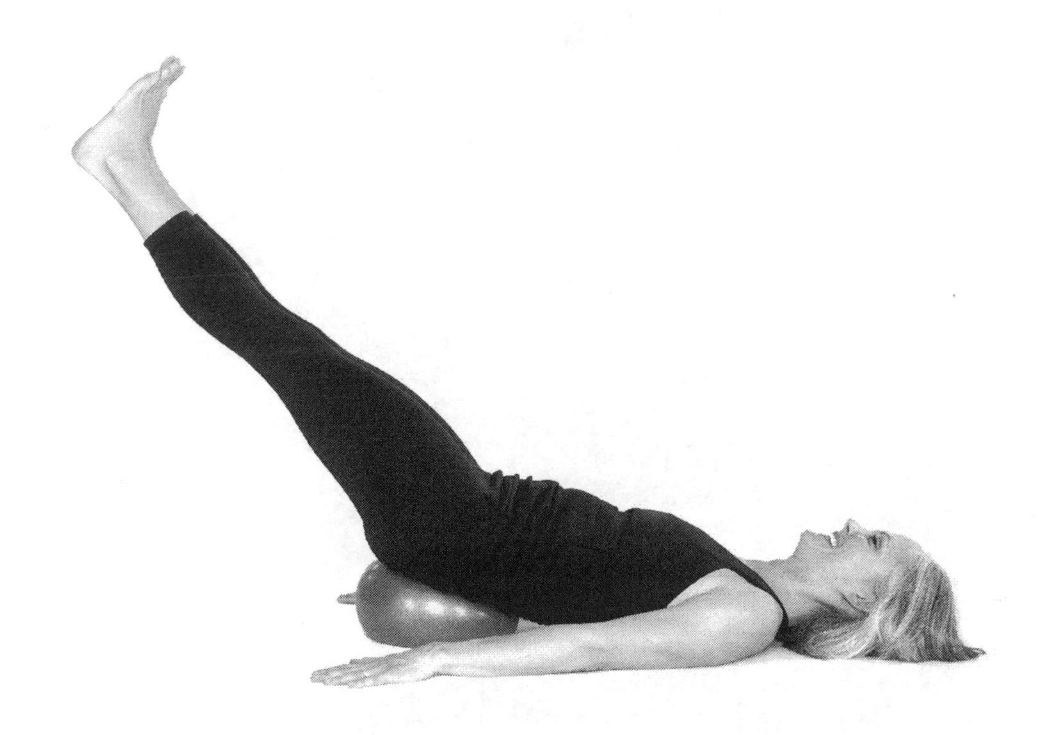

Leg Extensions on the SPRI Ball

3x10 (That means 3 sets of 10, resting about 30-60 seconds between sets)

Lie on your back, placing the SPRI Ball under your tailbone. Extend your legs to the ceiling, flexing your feet as if you could stamp the bottoms of them on the ceiling. Draw your belly in, engaging your core, while pressing into the SPRI Ball. Slowly lower your heels to where the ceiling meets the wall and hold for one breath before drawing the feet back to the starting position. Keep pressing the back rib-cage down toward the floor. With control and steady breathing, repeat 9 more times to finish the first set.

3

Woggling

Erin's Edition:

When my daughter was a baby, I started running. It began as a way to simply get out of the house. I'd strap my daughter, Izzie, into the jog stroller I inherited from Andra and off we'd go. What I quickly discovered was that, even though I enjoyed it, my body was not designed for fast, pounding movements. I then created what I term "woggling."

Woggling is faster than a walk and slower than a jog, but there's still a little "wiggle" in your booty. My husband David (a seasoned long-distance runner) calls it "the zombie shuffle". And while it is slow, there is no shamble! I taught Andra to woggle, and we have shared this awesomeness with countless women who also thought they couldn't run. We have woggled through deep depression, job changes, home construction, and the stress of raising tweens and teens.

If you can walk, you can woggle!

How to Woggle

Studies show that 60-80% of runners are injured yearly, mostly from repetitive use injuries (basically, too much pavement pounding with poor body mechanics). How do you run injury-free? By running softly, from your core, and with perfect biomechanical posture.

What's perfect biomechanical posture? In yoga, we call it tadasana, the mountain pose. If you want to run, get thee swiftly to a good yoga class and learn how to stand correctly first!

How to do Tadasana

Find a neutral spine that honors the natural curvature of your back. From the side, you should be able to draw an imaginary line from the ear to the ankle, passing through the shoulder and middle hip. The heels should be in line with the femur bone and the outer edges of the feet should be parallel to the sides of your mat. This foot alignment prevents you from pronating ("flat-footed," or collapsing inward) or supinating (having too high an arch and too much pressure on the outer leg). The tailbone points toward the floor slightly and the lower ribs are pulled in toward your heart to activate the core. Engage the quadriceps muscles slightly to lift the kneecaps. This will help later when you start woggling, as women tend to have a lot of trouble with their patella (knee cap) not "tracking" as it should. Soften the muscles of your face and breathe deeply.

Mastered Tadasana? You're Ready to Woggle!

Woggling is at its very heart a moving mountain pose. You're looking for a 12-14 minute mile. Woggling is low impact and easy on your knees, as one foot is always on ground. Your feet should strike the ground directly under the hips, and you hit the ground on the midsole (ball of the foot), not on the heel! Your face and shoulders are relaxed and your head stays over your shoulders (ears are in line with shoulders, never forward of them). As you woggle, transfer your weight evenly and softly from one foot to the next.

The core drives your propulsion. The navel is slightly pulled in toward your spine and the lower, front ribs - imagine that they "kiss" the heart at all times. Think about floating above the ground rather than bouncing. It's gentle, but it's still very challenging! This is appropriate cardiovascular training. Depending on your current fitness level, you should aim to work at no more than 55 -75% of your maximum heart rate.

Myth: Woggling will destroy your knees.

Truth: Woggling is no harder on your joints than walking. Since it's powered from a strong, stable core, the impact to your knees is minimal. The exception is if you are currently morbidly obese (based on medical standards). If you are morbidly obese, we suggest starting with weight training and gentle yoga to help rid the body of fat before you add exercises that ask you to weight-bear while moving. Every pound of fat you are over your body's "happy place" places up to 4 extra pounds of pressure on your joints. So if you are currently 25 pounds overweight, each step places 100 extra pounds of pressure on your knees.

If you can still carry on a conversation, but couldn't sing an entire song without getting "breathy", then your heart rate is elevated appropriately!

Andra's Addition:

The Art of Woggling

Have you ever looked at a runner as you whizzed past them in your car? Not just a glance so you don't hit them, but really looked at their facial expression and body posture? If you haven't, try it and you'll notice that most (not all, mind you, but most for sure) look utterly miserable. Their face is distorted with anguish and pain as if they're running in an actual zombie apocalypse, trying desperately with every part of their body to run and escape from fast approaching undead brain-munchers! If you look closely enough, you can almost see the pack of zombies closing in on them.

Maybe that's a tad dramatic, but they do often look pretty uncomfortable. At least that's what my unscientific, entirely random on-going completely unfounded and disregarded personal study of runners absolutely confirms! From my comfy heated car seat, most of them look uncomfortable.

Perhaps my assessment is a bit clouded, because for many years I desperately wanted to be a runner. I longed to both be and be seen as a runner. Certain that being a runner would solidify me as actually "in shape," I tried and failed many times to establish a running habit. I believed that if I could only become a regular runner, there would be no denying my physical prowess. And of course I would be proud and happy (with a dash of smug.) Along this misguided path, I enjoyed periods of success with much basking and periods of failure laden with nagging hip and knee aches, frustration and plenty of negative self-talk.

Until one day, the roller coaster stopped looping. A close friend had entered into a six-month biweekly personal training contract with a new facility in town. Her three kids were all finally school age and she was trying to get in better shape. Great, right?

Yes, except that her workout buddy quit her part of the contract with five months to go and left my friend hanging with the remaining contract's balance. She contacted me and asked me to fill in to cut the cost, just until it was up for renewal. It was right after my kid's drop-off time for school, she knew I valued exercise, would pay for it and most likely help her out. Great, except remember that smug part?

As it should happen, I was in a brief but successful part of the running loop and really adhering to a routine. I was training for an upcoming run and down in a running groove! I thought to myself, "I don't need to go to a personal trainer because I'm already in shape." Despite this arrogance, I decided to help her out because she was trying hard and a really good friend. Fast forward to our first session the following week.

We're beginning with some basic sit-ups and all of a sudden, the roller coaster grinds to a halt and my worldview is shattered. Well, maybe not my worldview, but certainly my view of me! And why? Because I could not do one single solitary sit-up. I am absolutely serious. Not. One. Fucking. Sit-up.

Remember how I arrogantly view myself as completely in shape and not needing the services of a personal trainer? If I was so in shape, then why couldn't I do a sit-up? I lost all sense of decorum and continued to writhe, struggle and strain red-faced with spittle flying to just…sit…up…one time!

In fact, I tried so hard that something actually popped inside my lower abdomen, frightening me enough to surrender, panting on the floor to the muffled sounds of my friend stifling her giggles! After a few seconds of bewildered pouting, I joined in laughing too.

To this day, I don't know what popped, but I am pretty sure it was my ego being forced to acknowledge that I had a floppy core. I couldn't do one blessed sit-up because my core was weak, genuinely weak. I had a physical weakness!

Following this realization, an internal tsunami of anger, frustration and negativity swirled around inside me with my inner monologue shouting, "for fuck's sake, what else can't I do? Where else am I weak? Why am I making myself run if it's not getting me in shape? What is happening to my body?" This continued until I grew weary of throwing fits and decided it was time to take action. I ditched the running schedule not because I had to but because I chose to. I had to make some muscles!

Sticking with the contract, I began to strengthen my core with the help of a personal trainer. Not just building a "6-pack" but really focusing on my entire trunk, front and back. As I worked each week, I began to notice my posture, daily movements and general views about fitness changing. The work was hard and my body was sore. I mean Advil and hot baths sore, please don't hug me sore, and I cannot get up off the toilet sore! But I stuck with it and started paying attention to what was going on inside my body.

I began to listen and focus on the inside instead of the outside. I didn't care how I was perceived - I wanted to be strong from the inside out. I no longer defined being in shape as a finished goal but gradually started to view it as a process to be continually refining.

With my attitudes about my body and exercise changing, I wanted to incorporate more exercise into my life instead of feeling like I should incorporate more exercise into my life. Having done yoga in my thirties, I added a weekly class. Growing up as a competitive swimmer, I began swimming some laps at the local indoor pool. I even began running with my neighbor, Erin (you know, her in the yoga poses).

Except we weren't running…we were doing this slow shuffle she'd christened "woggling." Woggling? What in the world was woggling? Well, everybody knows that woggling is an intelligent alignment-based sustainable cardio movement. Remember the uncomfortable joggers fleeing the zombies from the beginning of this tale? The ones who looked so miserable? Well, wogglers don't look like that because they aren't uncomfortable. Their bodies are in proper alignment - they are propelling themselves forward from their strong core and landing on the balls of their feet with soft knees and hips at a slow and sustainable speed. Wogglers won't be winning any races, but they will be finishing them! And without aching hips and knees!

To serious runners, woggling seems like a waste of time. To master the art of woggling, you must let go of some running attachments. As I've already stated, you won't win any races except the be-active-in-your-golden-years one if that's important to you. Woggling is about the journey, not the finish. That's why wogglers look more at ease and less miserable than the joggers I observe. It's about enjoying the intelligent alignment-based sustainable cardio movement that's propelling you forward instead of about doing it as fast as you can and checking fitness off your to-do list.

Most people aren't designed to run six days a week and we disregard structural weaknesses resulting in discomfort and injury. Believe me, I know and lived this! Now, I woggle when the weather is nice once or twice a week at the most.

Why so rarely? Because woggling is one part of my exercise portfolio! I don't burn out or have nagging injuries and I'm not attached to keeping anything other than my hips, knees and overall body strength. And I never feel like the stale breath of zombies down my neck!

Walking is Great Too!

Woggling not your fave? No worries. Walking is a fabulous way to move your body. It improves posture, strengthens your heart and lungs, increases blood flow to your brain, improves your breathing capacity, lowers stress, and promotes restful sleep. It has been said that every minute of walking lengthens your lifespan by one extra minute. So rather than thinking, "I don't have time for a thirty minute walk", think "if I walk for thirty minutes now, I gain an extra thirty minutes of my life to do something amazing!" Most people walk about 65,000 miles in their lifetime - that's three times around the earth!

Make it value-added by eschewing the treadmill and getting outside. According to studies, the closer you live to nature, the healthier you're likely to be. There is a strong correlation between time spent indoors or in polluted cities and diseases including cardiovascular, respiratory, and neurological conditions. And try to go outside in the morning. People who load up on light exposure at the beginning of the day are most likely to have a lower body mass index, because the blue light waves of early morning balance our circadian rhythms (which tell our brains when we are both hungry and full).

Nature is the perfect place to move your body. Ever notice how your mind zones out totally on the treadmill or spinning bike? You are forced to be mindful when hiking or cycling outdoors (lest that unseen tree root up-end you). Fresh air and natural movement are our birthright and so often squandered or taken for granted. So lace up and get outside!

Better yet, skip the shoes and go barefoot if you have a safe place to walk. We receive electrons from the earth that make us healthier!

Grounding the body allows negatively charged antioxidant electrons from the Earth to enter the body and neutralize positively charged free radicals in inflamed areas.

Sounds crazy, right? Scientists have actually documented a reduction in inflammation using MRI while measuring blood chemistry and white blood cell amounts before and after grounding. What they found is that the electrical currents rooted in the earth's layers make the ground under our feet a huge antioxidant! Plus, going barefoot will strengthen and stretch the muscles and fascia of the foot, creating wonderful trickle up benefits to your knee and hip joints.

Erin's Edition:

Into the Woods

I've always loved the woods. I was raised in the forest, my youth spent climbing trees and catching crawdads in the creek behind our house. Those woods offered endless backdrops for our imagination - the trees and rocks became pirate ships, rockets, and, most often, the Death Star (this was, after all, the 70s and my older brother always got his way).

Even now, there is no balm to my soul like the loamy smell of the under-canopy. Lying on the forest floor, with shafts of light piercing the leaves like scattered diamonds, it's easy to connect to Source.

Everyone rhapsodizes about the ocean. And sure, I love the ocean too. But I wouldn't choose to live there. The beach is too turbulent, with its roiling waves, strong winds, and pounding storms. There isn't enough stillness. My default setting is movement, a body always in motion. The beach energizes me, but ultimately makes me feel untethered, like I could be washed away on the next tide.

The woods offer just the right balance of movement and stillness. The yang of the babbling brook is tempered by the yin of the strong, silent trees. The birdsong is a backdrop rather than a noise that demands attention. The rocks and trees buffer from strong winds and rainstorms. Once you step into the trees, everything smells fresher and more real.

I'm especially obsessed with a local area called the Red River Gorge. When you stand barefoot on sandstone, you stand witness to eons of history. It helps to put things into perspective. When my troubles seem insurmountable, I like to stand on the rocks, knowing they will quickly erase all evidence of my presence. Carve your name into the top of the rock that forms Kentucky's Natural Bridge and, eventually, even that will be blown clean. That same gentle wind can sometimes scrape clean the sky, revealing a blue only Kentuckians are privy to. It's magical.

Scientists like Richard Louv, who wrote the seminal book *Last Child in the Woods*, worry that children are spending less time in nature, with the result a wide-range of behavioral disorders. Studies show that as screen times in children have accelerated, visits to America's National Parks have declined.

We can draw the conclusion that if less time in nature is bad for our children, it's equally harmful to adults. Walking outside elevates the experience in so many ways. Walking is cheap, and available to almost everyone. Put the two together for added value. Being outside enlivens your senses, creating an opportunity for mindfulness not available on the treadmill. It sharpens your senses and clears your mind in a way walking on the street cannot. Our connection to nature is so important and needs to be nurtured.

How Much Is Enough? The Devil That is Overtraining

How much cardio is enough? Of course, this answer is different for each person. But there are a few guidelines. Two to three miles twice to three times a week is perfect for us. You might need more or less. But err on the side of less.

Yes, we just gave you permission to skip a workout! Are you thinking we've lost our minds? There is a widespread misperception about cardio and fat loss. Most people think that, to get skinny, you need to slash your calories and do at least an hour of high-intensity cardio each day. In reality, too much cardio engages that catabolic state, where your muscle cells are dying off more quickly than they are being replenished. This muscle loss will not only reduce strength, but it will also slow down your metabolism! This is a double whammy if you're looking to burn fat and build muscle!

We believe 45-60 minutes of low to moderate intensity cardio is appropriate a few times a week. Any more is likely counterproductive (especially if you aren't consuming enough protein to support that caloric outflow).

Cardio is fine and we love our woggles, but flexibility and

strength training is king when it comes to longevity!

4

Do Something You Love

There is no one exercise that satisfies every goal. Your body will eventually adapt to the same form of exercise and routine and you'll plateau in your strength and flexibility gains.

Challenge your body by changing it up and you'll keep progressing in your fitness goals.

Periodically changing things like how much weight you're lifting or how quickly you are walking will help you get lasting results while minimizing risk of injury. Doing the same thing over and over slows your progress and sets you up for repetitive use injuries.

So every week, move your body in a way that you love. Try something new. Move out of your comfort zone. Ride a bike. Hike a trail. Try Zumba. Dance in your living room. Whatever floats your fitness boat! Just do something that isn't yoga, resistance training, woggling, or walking so you continue to grow stronger and happier.

> **Journal Prompt**: Are you someone who struggles to enjoy movement? You know it's good for you, but you just don't love it? We think you just probably haven't

found the right form of exercise! To decide where to start, journal about your exercise history.

When was the last time you really enjoyed moving your body (and, yes, sex totally counts). When was the last time you felt strong? Beautiful? Free? Are you impulsive or more goal-oriented? Do you need extrinsic motivation, like a coach or a specific goal to work towards? Do you prefer to be alone or in the company of others? Inside or outside? Music or silence? Morning or evening? Do you consider yourself a leader or follower? Do you like to try new things or prefer the tried-and-true?

The answers to these questions can help you choose activities you'll stick with. Using your answers, generate a list of activities that resonate with you and activities that do not. Stay away from those things that set you up for failure. We are all motivated by vastly different things, so spend some time getting to know you.

PART FOUR
REST

We believe self-care and true rest are the most-often-neglected parts of a wellness program. Self-care is not indulgent or selfish. It's a necessary priority that allows you to feel calm and whole so that you can share your gifts with those around you. As care givers, we are focused on the needs of others so much we often neglect ourselves.

Self-care is a necessity for busy women. We need to draw energetic boundaries or our lives can become a never-ending chore of cleaning and driving. There is always a dish to wash, a pet to feed, a child who needs a ride somewhere. It's imperative that we carve out time each week just for ourselves so that we have the energy to take care of our loved ones.

Most people think that in order to become healthy they must lose weight. Actually the opposite is true. In order to lose weight, one must become healthy.

We all know that gym rat that runs mile after mile on the treadmill and eats next to nothing but cannot lose weight. Maybe they are thin, but they do not look healthy. Why not? Shouldn't a punishing workout regimen and a 1,200 daily calorie diet result in a fit, healthy body? Not necessarily. These are the Skinny Fat people.

For the answer, we must understand how the autonomic system (ANS) works and how we can balance it. It's about to get all science-y again, but bear with us.

The ANS is what runs our body behind the scenes - it regulates our heartrate, respiration, immune system, body temperature, organ functions, and on and on. It is made up of the Sympathetic Nervous System (SNS), which is the "fight or flight system" and the Parasympathetic Nervous System (PNS), which is the "rest and digest system".

The SNS is catabolic, while the PNS is anabolic. They generally have opposite functions. When we are under stress, the sympathetic system engages with our heart rate accelerating, our breath becoming faster, and the adrenal glands releasing cortisol so that we can either run away from or fight whatever is threatening us. If we are chronically stressed, that increases the load on the sympathetic system as well.

The sympathetic system is catabolic, meaning it breaks down muscle tissue due to high cortisol levels. High-intensity physical exercise is also sympathetic in nature - the heart rate goes up, respiration goes up, body temperature goes up, and cortisol is released into the blood stream.

The parasympathetic system tries to balance the SNS by slowing the heart rate and respiration back down, bringing blood back to the digestive tract, and repairing tissue damage.

When we are deeply resting, we enter an anabolic state where we are building new cells faster than cells are dying off.

Deep sleep gives the PNS the time it needs to repair cells and build muscle. But any restful activity will help to balance the ANS, thus making it easier to build muscle, sleep deeply, and lose weight.

We don't want you to work harder - we want you to work smarter and rest more!

Most people today have an overactive SNS. A dominant SNS results in depression, anxiety, toxic relationships, a poor diet, and sleep-deprivation.

This is where the REST comes in. REST refers to any self-care program that balances your ANS.

Remember epigenetics, the study of how our environment alters our gene expression? When we're under chronic stress and constantly in a catabolic fight or flight response, our DNA reacts with our RNA to produce certain proteins that are associated with not only those dreaded "lifestyle diseases," but also with insomnia, migraines, acne, irritable bowel syndrome, and mood disorders.

But engage the rest and digest system and the proteins produced in your body encourage a peaceful mind, steady heartbeat, and balanced hormones.

Every week, engage the rest and digest system in these four ways. Follow the Four!

1. Deep Sleep
2. Restorative Yoga
3. Self-Care
4. Nurture Your Social Connections

1

The Power of Deep Sleep

Man is refreshed not by the quantity but by the quality of sleep. ~George Gurdjieff

Deep sleep is the magical time when the body does most of its repairs. When we snooze, body temperature, heart rate, and blood pressure plummet to conserve energy. Then, the body releases growth hormones that repair all the cellular damage we did while awake. People who regularly get less than 6 hours of sleep each night have a 50% increased chance of viral infections, heart disease, and stroke. They aren't getting enough deep sleep to build new, healthy cells. The average adult needs seven to eight hours of sleep per night, but studies indicate that over 40% of Americans get less than that.

Myth: You need 8 uninterrupted hours of sleep to reap the benefits.

Truth: If you've made it this far in the book, then you know that each of us is metabolically different. The "perfect" amount of sleep is different from person to person. It is part of your wellness journey to figure out what amount supports the best you. You owe it to yourself and those around you to figure this out.

When we sleep, we go through four to five sleep cycles, each lasting about 90 minutes. Each cycle contains four phases: three phases of non-Rapid

Eye Movement (NREM) and one phase of Rapid Eye Movement (REM). During these phases, the brain is actively storing memories and doing some light handyman chores around your bod.

Lack of sleep makes us fat! Chronic sleep deprivation causes the body to produce less leptin, a hormone that reduces appetite, and more ghrelin, a hunger-stimulating hormone produced mostly in the stomach.

When you're exhausted, your brain sends signals that say you are constantly famished and never truly full, no matter how much you eat!

Studies show that women eat more calories on days when they sleep fewer hours the night before. Not good!

If you are chronically sleep deprived, getting real rest may require drastic changes. Firstly, let's talk about the bedroom. Make the bedroom an oasis of rest. The bed is for sex and sleep only! Maybe some light reading between the two, but that's it. Watch TV in another room. Send children to sleep in their own beds. Keep the temperature on the chillier side and use covers to regulate your body temperature. Remember not to drink caffeine after noon.

Banish the electronic devices from the bedroom! No ipads, iphones, or Kindle fires. Studies indicate that nighttime exposure to the blue light from these devices interrupts the production of melatonin. Deep in your brain is a gland called the pineal. It is about the size of a grain of rice. But for such a tiny thing it plays an incredibly important role in how rested we are! It is the only endocrine gland in contact with the outside world. The pineal is way back in the middle of the brain, but it can sense light much like a security light does. Even blind people have this function!

Melatonin is secreted here to regulate the body's circadian rhythm (our wake/sleep cycle). So when the rods and cones in your eyes see a screen late at night, the pineal gland thinks it is still daytime and tells the brain not to release melatonin. If there is no melatonin release, there is no sleepy time! We have even gone so far as to use electrical tape to cover every single light in our bedrooms (the tiny light on the thermostat, humidifier, even the sound machine)!

Treat yourself to really nice pillows, high thread count sheets, and maybe a diffuser with lavender essential oils (the scent of lavender is calming to the ANS). You are worth it! Turn off the light and rise about the same time each day to keep your circadian rhythms happy. You may sleep one extra hour on the weekends, but maintaining a regular sleep/wake schedule helps you sleep well over time. How much sleep you need to feel your best is about 80% genetic - we are each unique in this regard. Be mindful of how you feel with less or more and figure out the perfect amount for you!

Erin's Edition:

Discover Your Sleep Equation

After I had a baby, I started experiencing hormone-induced insomnia. It was the worst! I'd turn in at 9:00 pm and wake up at 1:00 am ready to take on the day. I'd toss and turn and fall back asleep around 3:00 am for another few hours. I was exhausted and had terrible brain fog all the time. I got a virus and couldn't get well for about 6 weeks. I gained back the 10 pounds I had lost while breastfeeding. I was emotional and cried at the drop of a hat. I tried sleep aids, but didn't like how groggy and out of it I felt the next day.

I was a librarian before I became a yoga therapist, so I knew how to find the research to help. I'm happy to report that I overcame the insomnia and sleep deeply 90% of the time now. For me, a dark room and a sound machine make the perfect environment. I take 1 mg of melatonin (any more and I have intense, scary dreams) and spray magnesium on my belly before bed. I like to turn the light off at 9:00 pm, sleep deeply, and awaken without an alarm around 5:00 am each day. Figuring out the magic equation for my sleep was so worth the effort!

Alcohol and Sleep

Andra's Addition:

Do Drinkers Dream of Drunken Sheep?

Ever drink at night and wake up feeling sluggish and unfocused? Or wake up way earlier than you needed to and couldn't get back to sleep? That's because a good night's sleep doesn't mix with late-night alcohol consumption.

My husband, Travis, enjoys a bourbon nightcap, occasionally. Let me clarify that he is certainly a moderate drinker and in all honesty someone who began consuming alcohol in his middle 30s. So by no means a heavyweight drinker, but we are from Kentucky and he does enjoy sampling local bourbons! Interestingly, we began to see a pattern emerge. We noticed that on most nights that he has a nightcap before bed, he wakes up at a 4am and is unable to go back to sleep. This of course, makes for an exhausting next day! We also noticed that this never happens to me. Why is that? Is Travis just a crappy sleeper and sleep is yet another area that I am superior? Sadly for me, no!

Believe it or not, there's actually something physiological happening. After thinking of our own drinking patterns and researching a bit, Travis and I learned that bedtime alcohol induces sleep during the first half of the night, but wrecks it during the second half of the night, preventing REM (Rapid Eye Movement) sleep. REM sleep is the good stuff where dreams occur and true restoration happens.

When we drink too much late at night, we interfere with that process thus causing a restless night's sleep and a sluggish next day. According to research by Christian Nicholas and Julia Chan at the University of Melbourne, alcohol use before bed causes competing brain activity during the second half of the night, resulting in poor sleep. "When you see alpha activity alongside delta activity during sleep, it suggests there might be some kind of wakefulness influence that could compete with the restorative nature of delta sleep," Chan says. This is OK occasionally, but clearly not a good idea routinely.

So why does this not happen to me? Well, it is nothing special as I was hoping for, but actually a simple usage pattern. As we've already established, I'm a total lightweight when it comes to drinking. I consume a delicious craft beer with dinner most nights. That being all I can handle and prefer, I don't partake in a bourbon nightcap. Because my alcohol consumption is much earlier in the evening, my body has processed the alcohol by bedtime and so it's off to REM dreamland for me. Give yourself at least an hour or hour and a half of not drinking before you hit the sack. This will increase your chances for a great restoring hibernating-bear-type slumber!

Now please don't get us wrong - we aren't about to give up alcohol and we aren't about to suggest that you should. We are just asking you to keep your alcohol use within the moderate category and don't regularly drink too late at night for the benefit of your own health and longevity. What exactly is moderate alcohol use? Well, we're glad you asked! It's probably less than you think and it's different for men and women.

According to the Mayo Clinic, moderate alcohol use is one drink a day for women of all ages and two drinks a day for men younger than 65.

Examples of one drink include:

- Beer: 12 fluid ounces
- Wine: 5 fluid ounces
- Distilled spirits (80 proof): 1.5 fluid ounces

Why are men's recommended amounts greater than those for women? Well, I wondered that too. There's tons of information and a quick Google search can clear up misconceptions. It's unfair, but basically, women absorb alcohol differently than men for a variety of physiological reasons:

1. Men dilute alcohol easier. Women have less body water than men and therefore the same amount of alcohol consumed by men and women of the same stature results in a greater concentration of alcohol in the blood for women. We get drunk faster! Make sure your daughters understand this before heading off to college!

2. Women have less of the alcohol-processing enzyme dehydrogenase in the liver. So consuming the same amount of al-

cohol as a man is less efficient for women and more detrimental (we had to give men something at which to excel!).

3. Monthly hormonal changes affect intoxication levels (those damn hormones show up everywhere, even in alcohol processing).

It's easy to think that consuming alcohol at night makes you sleep better, however it's just the opposite. Also, chronic and excessive over-drinking is just harder on women's fabulous bodies. So please be moderate in your alcohol consumption. Enjoy whatever kind of alcohol you prefer but take care of your precious body by prioritizing its health and sleep!

The end! ZZZZZZZZzzzzzzz......

> **Journal Prompt**: Another common obstacle to deep sleep is racing thoughts and worries, especially if you get in bed late. Your mind falls into a spiral of pessimistic thoughts. You worry you won't be able to fall asleep. Then you worry you won't feel well tomorrow. Then you worry about the project due and how you'll afford to send your kids to college and what you'll do if your spouse dies and you're left a widow. The longer you think, the more dire your thoughts become. Sound familiar? One solution is to spend a few minutes journaling before bed. Sometimes the simple act of writing down our worries can allay our fears. Studies show that college students suffering from insomnia gained more quality sleep time after journaling for 15 minutes each night for a week.

Try it! First, write down the exact transcript playing in your mind, then read it back to yourself. It won't take long to notice how you write down the same worries night after night. The act of writing them down helps to release them from your mind - you'll feel lighter after unburdening them.

As you close your journal each night, take a long, audible exhale. Let the sound of your breath indicate that those worries are "put away" for the night. Now sleep tight!

Magnesium

Have you ever wondered why you sleep so soundly at the beach? Firstly, your stress levels are probably pretty low because you're on vacation. Then, you have the sound of the waves lulling you to slumberville.

But did you know that the dip you took in the ocean earlier in the day probably has even more to do with it? The ocean is a great source of magnesium. For hundreds of years, people had appropriate levels of magnesium in their bodies just by eating plenty of vegetables. But in the last few decades, over-farming has stripped almost all of the magnesium from our soil, so it is almost impossible to get enough magnesium just from our diet.

Scientists calculate that almost 40% of Americans are deficient in this vital mineral. This is a real detriment to your sleep. Magnesium is responsible for over 350 enzyme reactions in your body. It plays an important role in hydration, muscle relaxation, energy production and the deactivation of adrenaline. So if you're deficient, your brain literally cannot power itself down at night! Try spraying topical magnesium on your skin before bed.

Practice Left Nostril Breathing

This calming pranayama (breathing) technique is known as chandra bhedana. It slows the heart rate and lowers the blood pressure after only two minutes. Lie in bed on your right side, with a pillow or bolster under the left knee. Cover the right nostril with your thumb and extend the fingers out. Then take 10 or 20 deep breaths out of your left nostril.

2

Restorative yoga

Myth: If I sleep well at night, I don't need to practice restorative yoga too.

Truth: Your brain waves are slower when practicing restorative yoga than when you're going about your day. But they are slightly more active than when you are sleeping, which means you can actually be aware that you are relaxed. This leads to a deeper, more profound relaxation.

The goal of restorative yoga is not to stretch or to strengthen. The goal is to truly let go. Restorative poses help to engage the relaxation response, balancing the nervous system, improving immune function, and accelerating digestion. It sets the whole body up for deep healing, growth and repair. And I bet you won't be surprised by now to learn that people who practice restorative yoga report longer, deeper sleep!

These yoga poses are completely supported with props so that we don't have to strain to be in or stay in them, allowing us to drop into a deep yogic rest. We try to be as passive as possible in order to release, entering into a space in which we can let go of all the layers of who we aren't in order to drop deep into who we are. These postures reset your brain from all of the processing it does all day long.

Because they are supported, you can comfortably stay in restorative postures much longer than traditional yoga asana. For the perfect practice, try all of the following, staying in each pose for about 10 minutes. This sequence includes a backbend, forward fold, twist, hip opener, and inversion.

To access restorative yoga videos with Erin and Andra, visit www.theOMplace.net.

Erin's Edition:

Drive Your Legs Up the Wall

If the energy scale goes from 1 to 10, where 1 is a rainforest sloth and 10 is a jack rabbit that just drank a red bull, my baseline is about an 8. I am a bubbly, highly energetic person. I normally pop out of bed an hour or so before the alarm sounds, smiling and ready to tackle my day.

Andra likes to say that I get more done before 8:00 am than most people accomplish all day, because by then, I have meditated, woggled, done a little yoga in the sauna, returned some emails, posted on social media, and made my breakfast shake. I talk fast, eat fast, and am so enthusiastic about life that I often exhaust those around me. David says that everyone in the world is a flashlight and I am one of those 15 million candle power flashlights that fireman use to shine through the thickest smoke. I burn hot and bright. So restorative yoga is something I resisted for a long time. While I intellectually understood its importance, it just isn't my natural inclination to choose stillness over movement.

In the winter of 2013, I got sick. I woke up one day with body aches and extreme exhaustion. I assumed I had the flu and just stayed in bed. Three days later, I felt no better. A week later, I was still worn out, that "so tired you could sleep on the median in rush hour traffic" exhaustion. I was swabbed, poked, and prodded. Low iron and vitamin B, no surprise there since I hadn't eaten in a week, but the tests couldn't pinpoint anything specific. I tested negative for strep, mono, the flu, and fibromyalgia. My doc finally diagnosed me with a "superbug" and told me to wait it out.

I was sick for three straight months. My joints ached, I was exhausted all the time, and I gained weight, even though I had no appetite (talk about unfair)! I had terrible brain fog that no amount of sleep would clear. I was unable to remember names, phone numbers, and basic vocabulary words. It felt like having a migraine in every part of my body. For the first time in my adult life, I didn't exercise at all. In the yoga classes I led, I just sat on my mat at the front of the room and led class. I cried a lot, slept a lot, and spent in inordinate amount of time lying on the bathroom floor moaning and feeling terribly sorry for myself.

I also started doing restorative yoga. It seemed I would have what my momma calls a "sinking spell" around 3:00 every afternoon. I noticed that if I put my legs up the wall and breathed deeply for 15 minutes, I felt better. Being ill is extremely dehydrating to your muscles, so I was stiff all the time. Because you aren't using energy to support your body's weight (the props do this work), restorative poses deeply relax the muscles and free the joints, leaving you more vibrant and energized. It also allows the body to shift into that anabolic state, supporting the body's ability to heal itself.

By the time the daffodils were pushing their bright yellow faces through the snow, my energy was starting to reemerge. I started eating again and taking walks in nature. By Memorial Day, my comeback was official. My eyes shone and my energizer bunny mentality returned. But my love and respect for restorative yoga had been cemented. To this day, I will put my legs up a wall - or headboard, tree, barn, car, airplane seat, or anything that will sit still - for a few minutes each day. It is my reset button for a great day, a mid-afternoon pick-me-up that works far better than an espresso or a bag of gummy bears.

Andra's Addition:

Add Some Exercise Diversity to Your Portfolio

Oh, restorative yoga! Truth be told, I used to view restorative yoga exactly the same as meditation - a colossal waste of time. I rationalized that I was already doing restorative yoga while I slept. I'm a great sleeper and there is simply no need to carve out extra time for this nonsense. How very wrong I was!

One day, I was both sore and tired and I actually participated in a restorative class. Well, let me back up. I was actually required to participate in a restorative yoga class during teacher training. At the end of yoga teacher training, there is a period known as "intensive week" where all prospective teachers are required to practice teach a yoga class. My class had 24 almost-teachers, so that averaged out to about six yoga classes a day for four consecutive days! Believe it or not, one can actually tire of yoga if participating in that many classes.

Nearing the end of the week, one of the would-be teachers noticed the physical/mental strain all this yoga was having on everyone and switched their game plan to a restorative class, rather than a normal yoga class. Even though I was required to participate, I really cannot express just how delicious the experience truly was. I was an instant believer and convert!

The magic of restorative yoga is that you put your body in poses that are supported by props. Therefore, you don't have to hold yourself in these positions. You are simply melting into the pose while being supported! When I practice even just a little restorative yoga each day, I notice that my body and mind are refreshed and better functioning for the rest of the day.

Restorative yoga is always incorporated in the yoga classes that I teach, sessions with my private clients as well as my own days /nights. I constantly encourage my clients and students to put themselves in a restorative pose at night after a long day. It's a perfect way to bring stillness and recuperation to a tired mind and body.

The specific reason it's so great is because it complements all the work performed by your body and mind each day. At the OM place, we are always preaching the benefits of "exercise diversity" which simply means doing different movements instead of the same form of exercise over and over. Restorative yoga should be one addition to our weekly exercise portfolios (sounds just like a financial planner, right?).

I completely understand the resistance to restorative yoga as wasting time when you could be getting things done. But I would argue that because you put yourself in restorative yoga for a few minutes, you actually get more done! Boom! How about that for blowing your mind? What can it hurt to give it a try?

Some Easy Home Restorative Yoga Examples

- Legs up the headboard or couch – Just lie on your back and place those legs on either the couch cushions or up your headboard. Allow your shoulders to fall open toward the ground and let gravity relax your hips. Breathe deeply for 10 good breaths or longer if you can. That's it! Move on with your day!

- Lie on your comfortable carpeted floor with the back of your shoulders over a bed pillow. Open your chest to the ceiling and breathe deeply 10 times, relaxing all your muscles on the exhale. Now, go get your shit done!

- Grab a pillow from your bed and place it on the floor. Sit with your legs together so your right hip is against the short end of the pillow. Placing a hand on either side of the pillow, simply fold over in a gently supported twist, laying your torso on the pillow. Rest the side of your face that is the most comfortable for your neck on the pillow. Breathe deeply here for 10 breaths, then switch to the other side by lifting up your body and placing the left hip against the pillow. Now, up and at them!

- Lie down on a flat, comfortable surface like a carpeted area or your bed. Bend your knees, placing the bottom of your feet on the floor hip-width apart. Lifting your hips, place a pillow under them and lower your hips back down resting on the pillow. You can keep your knees bent, or extend your legs out depending on how this feels to your lower back. Adjust the pillow as needed and relax your body, breathing deeply a few times. This should feel fantastic and be supportive to your lower back! You're ready to take on the world!

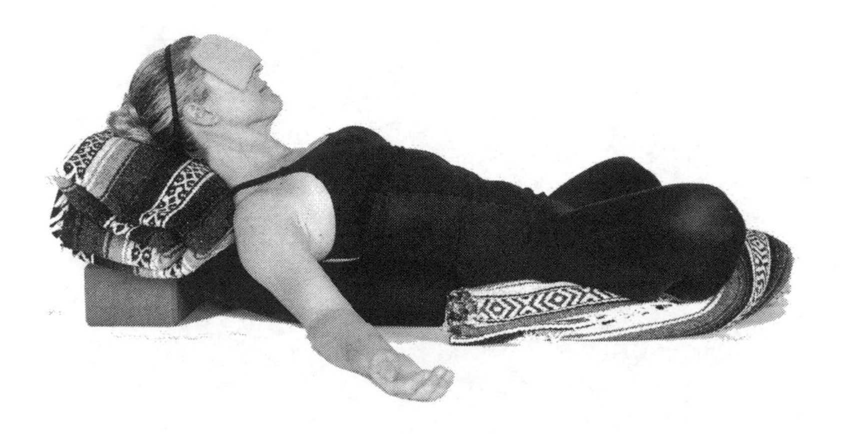

Supported Cobbler's Pose

Supta Baddha Konasana

What to do:

Place a bolster lengthwise on your mat. Place one folded blanket under your head at a preferred height. Roll the other blanket into a long tube. Sit so that the booty is on the floor, but the tailbone touches the short end of the bolster. Place the bottoms of your feet together and place the long roll over the feet, then wrap the ends under the outer legs. Lie back and rest for 5-15 minutes.

What it does:

Cobbler's pose is a fantastic way to open a tight chest (or wounded heart) and stretch the lower back and inner thighs. It allows the belly to soften, encouraging deep, relaxing breathing.

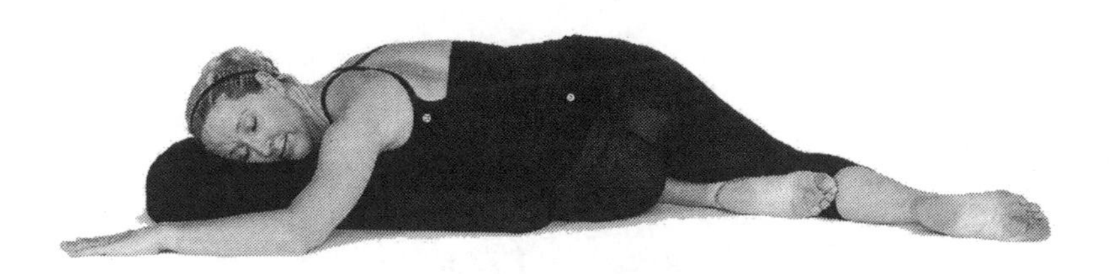

Bolster Twist

Salamba Bharadvajasana

What to do:

Place the bolster lengthwise on your mat and sit with the right hip touching the short end of the bolster, knees pointing to the left side of the room. Turn the torso so the belly rests on the bolster and the arms rest in a "goal post" shape on either side of the bolster. Head is facing either way - you can bring the left ear to the bolster or, if your neck is tight, simply rest the right cheek on the bolster. Rest for 3-5 minutes, then switch sides for the same amount of time.

What it does:

Twists help to nourish the discs between the spinal bones. Also, the internal organs are gently compressed during a twist. When the twist is released, fresh blood flows to those organs, carrying oxygen and nutrients to the tissues for healing.

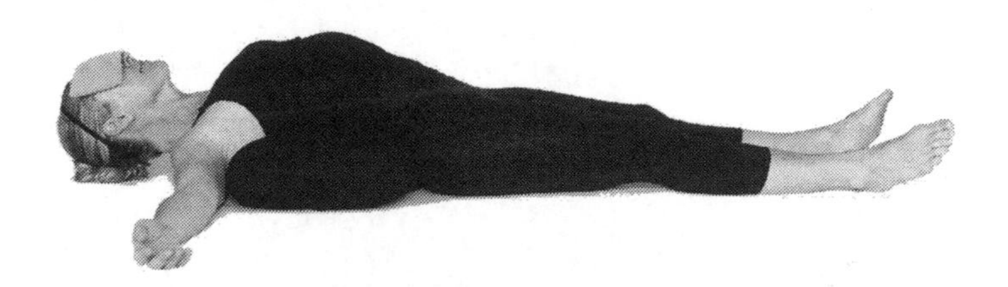

Supported Fish

Salamba Matsyasana

What to do:

Place a bolster sideways across your mat. Sit with your legs out long and your tailbone touching the bolster. Lie back and place a yoga block under your head. Let the arms rest in a "T" between the block and the bolster to further open the chest. If the low back gets cranky, either bend the legs or place a blanket under the hips to lessen the degree of the backbend.

What it does:

This heart opener is fabulous for countering all the hunching we do all day! All the texting, emailing, and driving we do rounds our shoulders forward and tightens the muscles of the front chest. This pose opens that tightness up and helps to relax the neck.

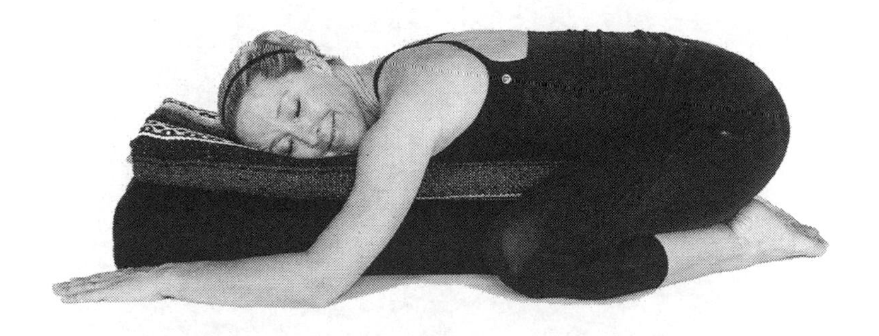

Bolster Child's Pose

Salamba Balasana

What to do:

Place a bolster lengthwise on your mat and stack 1-2 blankets on top. Kneel at one end with the knees wide, shins and feet resting on the floor. Lay the torso over the bolster, leaving ample space for the torso to stretch out entirely. Turn the head to rest on the bolster end. Adjust the blanket height, as needed. Rest for a few minutes, breathing across the back of your body.

What it does:

This forward fold gently stretches the spine and calms a frazzled nervous system very quickly. It is especially useful for high stress times in your life.

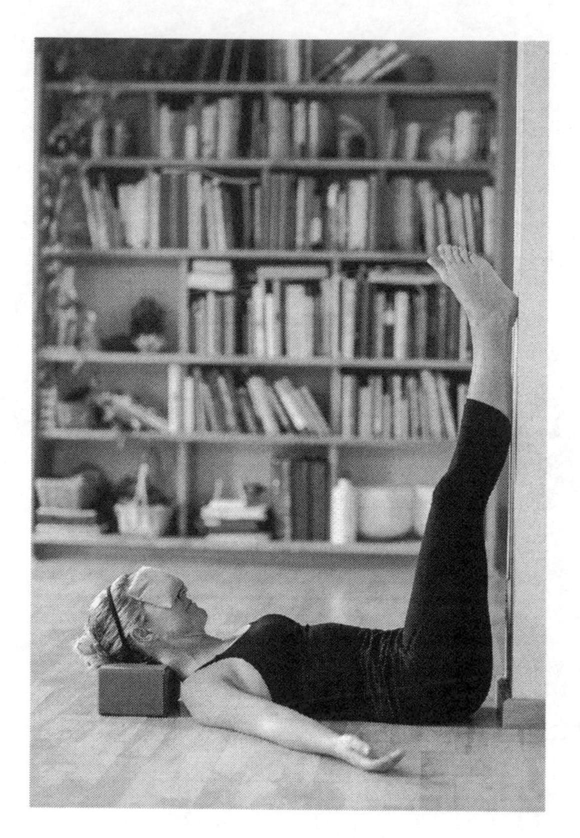

Legs Up The Wall

Viparita Karani

What to do:

Sit by a wall with your hips as close to the wall as possible. Spin the torso out into the middle of the room as you stretch your legs up the wall. Place a blanket or block under your head so that your forehead is in line with or higher than your chin. Rest the arms comfortable out to the sides. Breathe deeply here for 5-30 minutes.

What it does:

Inversions improve the circulation of blood and lymph. They calm the mind and lower the blood pressure. This is the perfect pose to practice at the end of the day. This is Erin's all-time favorite yoga pose.

3

Self-Care

By this, we mean carving out time each week to do something alone. Here are a few delicious ideas of ways to get your Alone-not-Lonely-on.

Bodywork

Virtually every culture throughout history has healed through the power of touch. Massage reduces stress, stimulates the lymphatic system, and eases painful conditions of all kinds. It is Erin's go-to self-care activity.

Infrared Sauna

Infrared saunas heat up the user's body rather than heating the air. It creates radiant heat from long light waves not visible to the eye. These rays penetrate more deeply below the skin than regular saunas, vibrating fat molecules to release toxins. It boosts circulation, lymph drainage, and the release of mucho toxins through sweating.

Roll it Out!

Use a therapy ball or foam roller to perform self-myofascial release (a fancy term for self-massage to release muscle tightness or trigger points). Fascia is the fibrous and collagenous structure that makes up 30% of our total muscle mass. Fascia has an appearance similar to a spider's web or a sweater. Healthy fascia is very hydrated and has a viscous, semi-fluid, elastic quality to it. Fascia is very densely woven, covering and interpenetrating every muscle, bone, nerve, artery and vein, as well as all of our internal organs. Think about a sandwich covered in saran wrap and how it holds all the sandwich parts together. That's fascia.

The most interesting aspect of the fascial system is that it is not just a system of separate coverings. It is actually one continuous structure that exists from head to toe without interruption. In this way, you can begin to see that each part of the entire body is connected to every other part by the fascia, like the yarn in a sweater. Fascia tightens as we age. This is a result of the habitual "propping" (how we hold our bodies throughout the day) as well as from the normal aging process.

By applying pressure to specific points on your body using a ball or roller, you are able to aid in the recovery of fascia and the surrounding tissues to return them to normal function. Normal function means your muscles and fascia are elastic, healthy, and ready to perform at a moment's notice.

Aromatherapy

Olfactory response is processed in the amygdala, the part of the brain connected to emotion. Basically, we process scent as an emotion before we process it as a thought. Scent-triggered memories are some of our strongest and most enduring. Lavender has long been the go-to scent for relaxation (it's used in the eye pillows at our yoga studio). Lavender can help calm the mind and body and has been used effectively to treat both insomnia and depression in many studies.

Neti Pot

This nasal irrigation device is beneficial for treating various sinus conditions using salt water and gravity. A neti looks like Aladdin's lamp. You fill them with warm salt water and pour into one nostril (it drains out the other). It thins mucous and helps flush out the nasal passages. Does pouring something into your nose make you nervous? You're not alone. Watch videos online to learn how to do it. It doesn't hurt at all and can be a lifesaver for those people with allergies and chronic sinus infections.

Soak in the Tub

One or two cups of cider vinegar added to a nice hot tub are all you need to rejuvenate. This is a really good bath for energy and it is fabled to help with urinary tract infections. Apple cider vinegar will help your body to become more alkaline - too much partying, alcohol, sugar, processed food and/or caffeine can make your body overly acidic. A 30-40 minute soak can help re-establish the balance.

Dry Brushing

The biggest organ in your body is your skin, accounting for about 16% of your body's weight. Dry brushing stimulates your lymphatic system and supports your body's inner cleaning. Start at the feet and brush in long strokes moving toward the heart. Make small circles around areas of lymph nodes (knees, groin, armpits, etc.)

Lie on the Couch with a Good Book

This is Andra's go-to when she's over-scheduled and overwhelmed. This low-stress activity has been shown to reduce stress levels by up to 68% in just 6 minutes! It strengthens the neural pathways in our brains to prevent age-related cognitive decline. Reading before bed has been shown to help you sleep more deeply when you do turn out the light.

Rebounding

Jumping on a mini trampoline is gentle on the joints but is fabulous for stimulating the lymphatic system. The alternation of gravity and weightlessness gently squeeze your cells. Hello, lymph flow!

Just Say "No!"

Sometimes "no" is the most positive thing we can say! Drawing your energetic boundaries is one of the best things we can do to practice self-care.

> **Journal Prompt**: What are some draining activities you'd like to say "no" to? Why do you continue to agree to them? Choose one thing from your list and develop an exit strategy for extricating yourself. It might help to practice the following line in front of the mirror. "Thank you so much for thinking of me, but that will not work for me right now". Say it politely, say it with a smile, but say it firmly. Don't explain further.

Erin's Addition:

Find Something That Fills Your Cup

As a teacher and writer, I spend a lot of time in verbal territory.

Working jigsaw puzzles engages a different part of my brain, helping me to stay sharp. A jigsaw puzzle has no deadline. I set one up on the rarely-used end of the table and work it as I feel called to. There's no beating that euphoric moment of placing the last piece in a 1,000 piece puzzle!

Andra's Addition:

My stress shows up as anxiety. It makes it hard to meditate or be still with my breath. So I prefer to use my hands to calm my nerves. Knitting is the perfect flow state. It only takes minutes to become so absorbed in my craft that my worries fall away. Studies have shown that elderly knitters had slower cognitive decline than their peers who just watched television and I don't know about you, but I want to be a sharp, sassy grandma!

Erin's Edition:

A Really Kick-Ass Pair of Jeans

Now, I realize how superficial this one sounds. But every woman deserves one garment that makes her feel absolutely amazing and nothing makes us feel sexier or more confident than a great pair of jeans. Finding that elusive perfect pair is harder than winning the lottery, but it's totally worth the effort.

Now I'm 5'1" with a really big booty (which I love, by the way). Junior jeans fit me in the length, but won't come up further than my knees. Petite jeans are too high-waisted. They scream "mom jeans" so loud I literally feel my ovaries shriveling up when I put them on. Not a recipe for sexy.

I ordered no less than 23 pairs of jeans from Zappos in the span of a few months on my quest for the perfect denim. Zappos, bless them, will let you buy and then promptly return anything you don't like, with free shipping both ways. This way, you can dim the lights in your room to that setting where you look alluring and attractive instead of simply exhausted.

You can drink wine, though be careful not to spill any on the jeans - I became the owner of a too-tight pair of DL1969 jeans this way! You can try on each pair with your favorite boots, flats, and heels. You can have a friend or husband there if you want. My husband is awful in this case, as he would think I look adorable and sexy in a full-body, Breaking Bad-style Hazmat suit. You want that friend who truly knows your body and understands the difference between "sexy tight" and "so tight you'll have to unbutton them to drive and forget eating anything in them."

My perfect pair is made by Paige. The four-way stretch means they fit more like yoga leggings than your old-school Levi's. Did I pay over $200 for them? I did. Was it worth every penny? It was, because I feel like a million bucks when I wear them. So when you crunch the numbers, I actually made money. That's just basic math!

Let's Talk About Sex, Baby

No section on rest would be complete without discussing the stress-buster known as sexual intercourse. The female orgasm is one of the quickest paths to a zen, flow state. When you're getting some play, your brain releases a rush of dopamine and oxytocin, two feel-good hormones that signal you to keep on doing whatever it is you're doing. At the same time, the part of brain that controls anxiety and fear shuts down. Talk about a win-win!

> *Myth: Women in their forties are no longer interested in sex.*
>
> *Truth: Hell no! We get just as hot and bothered as we did in our twenties, albeit maybe not as often. Our lives have just gotten busier, so it's harder to fit it in. And hormonal fluctuations sometimes complicate things. But it doesn't have to (as you'll find out later)!*

Regular sex is correlated with a stronger immune system, fewer migraines, better sleep, emotional balance, and stronger connections with your spouse or significant other.

So why then, in our 40s and beyond, do we seem to be getting less play? If sex in our twenties was for fun and sex in our thirties for procreation, what does sex in our forties and beyond look like? Well, it isn't that we don't love it (we do)! It's just that it takes a little more work at our age. Here are a few sex hurdles and how to clear them.

Lack of Privacy

There is no privacy because there are children in the house. Like, always. Everywhere. If they don't belong to you, they belong to the neighbor. How do you get your groove on with kids everywhere? You have to plan a little. This means relaxing the parenting rules and letting the kids watch another inane show on Disney Channel. Then locking the door (seriously, you have to lock that door). Maybe turn on a fan or the shower to drown out the noise. It's a hassle to plan, but it's well worth the trouble!

Disconnect Between Desire and Performance

You're turned on and into it, but your body isn't responding quickly enough. There is nothing worse than a disconnect between your brain and your vagina. In our 40s, declining estrogen levels means more vaginal dryness. Coconut oil to the rescue! Coconut oil is amazing as lube and can bail you out if the body can't keep up with the mind!

Your man also may have trouble keeping and maintaining an erection as he gets older. Seeing you looking hot may turn him on, but he might require actual stimulation to get an erection, which can be unnerving to both parties. That's where foreplay comes in. A few minutes of kissing, fondling, and massaging can make everything run more, uh, smoothly.

Poor Body Image

It doesn't seem fair that men seem to grow more handsome with age. But one advantage they have is that they seem to put less pressure on themselves to look a certain way. Hopefully, you're at an age where you have accepted and learned to love your shape. You certainly by this point know what you want in bed, so don't let a few lumps and bumps prevent you from getting some. He doesn't care if you have cellulite or didn't shave your legs. He's getting lucky and that is all the dinosaur brain in his penis cares about!

4

Nurture Your Social Connections

Now we're talking about fun, spirit-filling ways to spend time with people you love.

Spend Time with Friends

Try to do something every day that makes you laugh out loud! It changes the body's chemistry for the better and releases toxins. Psychotherapist Virginia Satir famously said, "we need four hugs a day for survival. We need eight hugs a day for maintenance. We need twelve hugs a day for growth." Hugging our loved ones releases oxytocin, a hormone that improves the immune system and lowers the levels of cortisol in the body.

Spend Time with Animals

Petting a dog or cat has been shown to engage the PNS quickly. Allergic to fur? Get a goldfish! Studies also show that watching an aquarium lowers stress levels.

Ask for Help!

Your loved ones want you to be happy, but they can't read your mind. If your self-care is lagging because you are overwhelmed, you need to learn how to ask for help. Write your spouse or children a list of things they can do to take the burden off you. When we get frustrated, we often find ourselves complaining about how we do everything around the house. But our loved ones often want to help - they are just unsure exactly how to provide support. So give them a detailed list of things they can do to lighten your load.

Andra has 12-15 index cards labeled with simple chores. She hands these cards out to her family each morning. When the chore is complete, they return the card to the basket on her kitchen table. She uses the cards over and over.

Sing, Dance, Cook

Make your meal preparation a party! Celebrate your healthy diet by turning on some music and dancing around your kitchen as you get dinner ready. We have no science to back this up, but we believe some good Motown can bring any human being out of a funk. Whisks make especially good microphones to belt out some tunes. Singing increases your lung capacity, improves your core strength, and helps you sleep!

> **Journal Prompt**: When was the last time you laughed so hard that your belly hurt? Who were you with? What happened? What is something or someone that makes you laugh, no matter how bad you're feeling? How can you cultivate this experience more in your life?

The Guidelines, Reviewed. Follow the Four!

Invite

Each day, spend five minutes doing one of the following:

1. Meditation
2. A Breathing Exercise
3. Journaling
4. Gratitude Attitude Training

Digest

As much as possible:

1. Replace soda with water, coffee, tea, or moderate amounts of alcohol
2. Replace refined sugar with protein
3. Replace artificial colors with true colors by "eating the rainbow"
4. Replace processed foods with real foods that have pronounceable ingredients

Move

Each week, try to perform each of these four activities once.

1. Yoga
2. Resistance Training
3. Woggle or Walk
4. Some Movement You Love

Rest

Every week, engage the rest and digest system in these four ways.

1. Deep Sleep
2. Restorative Yoga
3. Self-Care
4. Nurture Your Social Connections

Erin's Edition:

Too Tight, Too Loose

A few years ago, I started taking guitar lessons. Mr. Steve, my guitar teacher, is an aging hippie who writes poetry and smells of wood smoke and occasionally marijuana. He's patient and kind and idolizes Hank Williams. I adore him. The first thing he taught me to do is tune my instrument.

There's a story about a guitar player who once went to the Buddha for some advice about his life, which seemed to be spiraling deeper and deeper into chaos. The Buddha asked him what happened if he tuned his guitar too tightly. "The strings break," he answered. Then the Buddha wondered what happened if the instrument was strung too loosely. "Well, the sound won't come. You can only get a perfect note with a string that is not too tight and not too loose." The Buddha smiled and said nothing more.

Clearly, the point of the story is that our lives are a guitar. The process of fine-tuning never stops - you can't get to the perfect tautness and just stay there. Life requires some effort, but also some surrender to what is. We should constantly be making adjustments, retuning what works in an ever-present effort to find balance. In our thoughts, experiences, and choices, we should strive to be not too tight and not too loose. Where do we hold on when it isn't necessary? How can our lives be more about release and ease? How can we play loose, while holding onto our ideals?

Andra's Addition:

Give Yourself Some Space and Grace!

You know how your fingerprint is unique and no one in the universe has a fingerprint like yours? Or how your DNA is all you and no one can match it (unless you have an identical twin?) I see wellness exactly this same way - as unique to you as your DNA!

Erin and I have many similarities in our approach to wellness, but we also deviate in ways that serve each of us individually. For example, she's an early-riser and morning workouts are her preference. I, on the other hand, move a bit slower in the morning and prefer a later exercise time. Neither is right, or wrong, and it doesn't matter in the least. But what does matter, is that we each know what works for us and we stay within that construct. If you think about it, how could a weight-loss plan, fitness program or wellness guide designed by an individual person possibly work for everyone?

Have you ever listened to someone who has "figured it out?" It's a great way to solidify your wellness path because you will undoubtedly hear two things. Firstly, all the stuff that didn't work for them and second, how they really don't have anything figured out - they just know what works for them! You'll hear how they were as hungry and deranged as Cujo that weekend they tried a juice cleanse. Or how sluggish they felt when they drastically reduced their calorie intake. They'll take about the weight they gained back after stopping their restrictive diet. Or how their left shoulder ached all week after the Saturday morning TRX class taught by the perky millennial.

You get what I'm putting down here. But notice that in their descriptions, they are not bitter because they know this is actually the best thing about wellness. Discovering what doesn't work for you is imperative to establishing what does work! So all those "failures" are not failures at all, but discoveries of personal truths that let you put your wellness path together.

In addition to discovering what doesn't work, your Mrs. "Figured it Out" will also make an off-handed comment about how they don't have anything figured out. And she will laugh about it as if it's no big deal. And you will recoil in shock and horror.

But here's what she knows: none of us have anything figured out. And that's OK! You see, she knows that wellness is a moving target because everything around us is always changing. In order to keep ourselves on our wellness path, we have to be flexible. Like contortionist flexible, but only in our minds! We have to be willing to make an adjustment, shift our mindset, or change our approach, if something isn't working any more. We have to be willing to rip up that yellow-brick road and lay some new bricks to keep on our path. Just clicking the heels of those ruby slippers isn't going to work every time!

So what do you do? Be kind to yourself! Give yourself a break like you give everyone else in your life. If you miss a couple weeks of working out, that's OK. Just find your rhythm again by doing the kind of exercise that you prefer. Don't over-think it - just begin to move your body again!

Let your meditation practice go? Find you are missing that calm, grounding perspective you experience when you spend ten minutes sitting quietly with your morning tea before the busy house begins to stir? It's like riding a bike - find a quiet space, and spend a few minutes reconnecting with your inner self. You know how to do this!

Been spending the holidays living it up on Granny's peanut butter roll, Aunt Clare's cheese straws and two cocktail parties a week for the months of November and December? So what! The holidays will end and you can spend January not depriving yourself of good food, but eating cleaner. You know what to put into your body that will make it play like a finely-tuned piano!

Remember, all your previous work counts. Let me say that again – having a bad couple of weeks means nothing. All the work you did before the perceived "slump" counts for something! Own and accept that! Things are not perfect because our messy lives get in the way. Just realign, make a new plan, and start again with a forgiving and loving heart. Think of all the good work you have already done instead of beating yourself up about what you haven't done. Give yourself some space to be true to your unique needs and some grace when it's time to make an adjustment.

How Does She Do It?

So we just made it all sound really easy, right? It's not. We're told all the time how great we look and how easy it must be for us to stay in game-ready shape and how people wish they could do it too. But they can't because they are too busy. Or too tired. Or too poor. Or too...whatever.

Let's be perfectly clear. It's not easy. For anyone. But it does get easier with practice and habit. How do you create these habits? Mindfulness! Each and every day, you choose which habits you'll cultivate. There is no stopping point to wellness. It is an ever-changing undertaking.

We all have missteps, but every moment is a new opportunity to live mindfully and moderately. And we choose not to punish ourselves mentally for choices that are less than healthy. Everyone has weak moments where they abandon their meditation, or react with anger or frustration, overeat, or spend too many days without moving their bodies. Our success lies in our ability to forgive ourselves and move on, guilt-free. We fall off course, and we simply right ourselves again, like a compass that always points True North.

Remember Hara Hachi Bu, the Japanese idea of stopping eating when you are 80% full? We think Hara Hachi Bu is a great concept to utilize in your larger life. Nothing is all or nothing. Find your own True North, the ideals and concepts that best support the best you. Then 20% of the time, abandon those ideals completely.

Stay true, but keep it real. That's the secret.

Eat the cake. Skip a workout. Stay up late. Sing mental show tunes during your meditation. Play hooky from work. Tell a little white lie to carve out a few minutes to do something that is total and complete mindless fun.

Savor these moments. Then wake up and aim your inner compass toward your True North again.

What we're saying is that wellness isn't a secret obtained from an expert - wellness exists within all of us. You just need to tap into your own health and happiness. By learning to listen to your own common sense, you can begin to figure out what wellness path works for you specifically. What works for each of us will be different from person to person. Be willing to ride the changes of your life with ease and confidence and always be open to the next step in your wellness journey.

Girl, you so got this. You're amazing and beautiful and intelligent beyond measure. Now go build your life one delicious moment at a time.

Index

Index

Recommended Reading

INVITE

The Science of Happiness by Stefan Klein
Buddha in Blue Jeans: An Extremely Short Zen Guide to Sitting Quietly and Being Buddha by Tai Sheridan
Meditation: A Practical Guide to Making Friends with Your Mind by Pema Chodron
The Power of Now by Eckhart Tolle
The Book of Awakening: Having the Life You Want by Being Present to the Life You Have by Mark Nepo
The Art of Extreme Self-Care: Transform Your Life One Month at a Time by Cheryl Richardson
Healing Mantras: Using Sound Affirmations for Personal Power, Creativity, and Healing by Thomas Ashley-Farrand

DIGEST

The Eat Clean Diet by Tosca Reno
The Blood Sugar Solution by Mark Hyman, MD
The Yoga Body Diet by Kristen Schultz Dollard
Crazy, Sexy Diet by Kris Carr
The Beauty Detox Solution: Eat Your Way to Radiant Skin, Renewed Energy, and the Body You've Always Wanted by Kimberly Snyder, CN

Young for Life: The Easy No-Diet, No-Sweat Plan to Look and Feel 10 Years Younger by Marilyn Diamond
In Defense of Food by Michael Pollen
You: Staying Young by Michael Roizen, MD and Mehmet Oz, MD
Eating for Beauty by David Wolfe

MOVE

Your Best Body Now by Tosca Reno
The Women's Health Big Book of Yoga: The Essential Guide to Complete Mind/Body Fitness by Kathryn Budig
Tone it Up: 28 Days to Fit, Fierce, and Fabulous by Katrina Scott and Karena Dawn
Strong Is the New Skinny: How to Eat, Live, and Move to Maximize Your Power by Jennifer Cohen
Yoga: Ultimate Yoga Guide for Weight Loss, Stress Relief, and To Find Inner Peace! by Mia Conrad

REST

Sleep Soundly Every Night, Feel Fantastic Every Day: A Doctor's Guide to Solving Your Sleep Problems by Robert Rosenberg, DO, FCCP
Relax and Renew: Restful Yoga for Stressful Times by Judith Hanson Lasater
Restorative Yoga for Life: A Relaxing Way to De-stress, Re-energize, and Find Balance by Gail Boorstein Grossman
The Power of Rest: Why Sleep Alone Is Not Enough. A 30-Day Plan to Reset Your Body by Matthew Edlund, MD
The Women's Comfort Book: A Self-Nurturing Guide for Restoring Balance in Your Life by Jennifer Louden

Acknowledgements

Erin

Thanks to Rankin and Ruthi, my folks, for instilling in me a love for the written word in all its many forms and thinking my plan to live as a penniless librarian was a brilliant one.

Shout out to Andra, my sister wife, for seeing the real me and loving me anyway.

Props to the badass women of my Soul Tribe. You know who you are and I promise to never write about those nights. What happens on wine nights stays there.

And to David and Izzie for being the reasons. All of them.

Andra

To my parents, Zella and Vincent: Thanks for your steadfast love, constant cheerleading and infectious spontaneity. Also thanks for making me. I know you wanted more, but I've always been quite content with how it turned out!

Thanks to Erin for being the best friend, neighbor, teacher, boss, co-worker and co-author ever! But most importantly, thanks for pushing me when I need to be pushed, forgiving me when I can't keep up with you, loving me for who I am, and always making me laugh.

To my husband, Travis and kids, Connley and Harper: I am so blessed that you three sweet souls are all mine. Thanks for filling my life full of joy, laughter, patience and learning to share!

Acknowledgements from Both

While writing a book is often a solitary endeavor, publishing a book certainly is not. Special applause to Mike Ahern and Bryan Parnell of Cork & Bottle Publishing, who took complete drivel and turned it into a book even we wanted to read. This was no small feat.

It also takes a village to make us appear well put-together since, well, we aren't. Special thanks to Tina Carter for her beautiful photography and Jason Epperson for his mad visual guru skills.

Cheers to the practices of yoga, meditation, gratitude, and forgiveness for the opportunity to be ever more awake in our own miraculous existences. We would be insufferable without them.

About the Authors

Erin Smith, ERYT, CNT, MLS

Erin is a Warrior for Wellness. She has over 20 years and 5,000 hours of yoga teaching experience. She is the proud owner of the OM place yoga studio. She has a rich background in yoga, gymnastics, Thai Massage bodywork, nutritional consulting, neuromuscular therapy (NMT), and Meditation. Her interdisciplinary approach incorporates knowledge of anatomy, alignment, and various styles of movement therapy. She holds certifications from the Health Sciences Academy as both a Nutritional Therapist and a Sports & Exercise Nutritional Advisor. Erin's classes are influenced by her sense of humor, love of music, and wonder at the mystery of life. When she's not standing on her head, she enjoys being a wife, mother, woggler, dancer, reader, flower sniffer, guitar player, and wine drinker. She loves peonies, Mary Oliver, sushi, books that move her to tears, and crushing her bucket list. She looks forward to adding "published author" to her resume soon and plans to be a bird in her next life.

Andra Sewalls, ERYT, CPT, MLS

In 2014, Andra earned her 200-hour yoga teaching certification from the OM place and her personal training certification from the American Council on Exercise. She loves working with people to encourage healthy living and happiness through yoga and resistance training. In addition to her exercise certifications, Andra also has a Masters in Library Science from the University of Kentucky. Andra teaches OM Fit, True You and yoga classes at the OM place while also working with private clients. She is also the owner of Studio A, a home-based personal training and wellness service. When she is not teaching yoga, she enjoys spending time with her family, hiking, reading, taking amateur pictures and trying to make beautiful things! Andra loves Zac Brown, crafts, coffee with half and half, and her chickens (though she hates eggs with a passion)!

Andra and Erin have known each other most of their lives. They are in a long-term, committed exercise relationship that has evolved from pushing strollers to doing push-ups with their children. They are polar opposites and great friends. Andra likes sleeping late, country music, craft beer, and chana sag. Andra is a realist and an introvert. Erin is an early riser, loves acoustic folk, and is red wine and vegetable korma all the way. She is an eternal optimist and loves to be in front of a crowd. They are constantly struggling to balance being good wives, moms, friends, and business owners while changing the world one down dog at a time. Follow their missteps at #theOMplace #yogayoucanuse #studioA# selfcarenothealthcare

Made in the USA
Middletown, DE
11 August 2016